# HRT
# & the natural alternatives

# HRT
# & the natural
# alternatives

## Jan Clark

**TED SMART**

First published in Great Britain in 2003 by
Hamlyn, a division of Octopus Publishing
Group Ltd, 2–4 Heron Quays, London E14 4JP

This edition published for
The Book People Ltd,
Hall Wood Avenue,
Haydock,
St Helens WA11 9UL

Text copyright © Jan Clark 2003
Book design copyright © Octopus Publishing
Group Ltd 2003

ISBN 0 600 60853 0

A CIP catalogue record for this book is available
from the British Library

Printed and bound in China

10 9 8 7 6 5 4 3 2 1

**SAFETY NOTE**

While the advice and information in this book
are believed to be accurate and true at the time
of going to press, neither the author nor
publishers can accept any legal responsibility or
liability for any errors or omissions that may be
made. The reader should always consult a
physician in all matters of health and
particularly in respect of any symptoms which
may require diagnosis or medical attention.

# Contents

Introduction   *6*

Chapter 1 **Hormonal highways**   *8*

Chapter 2 **Hormone replacement therapy**   *22*

Chapter 3 **Alternatives to HRT**   *68*

Chapter 4 **Seeds of change**   *104*

Chapter 5 **Get moving!**   *122*

Bibliography   *139*

Index   *142*

Acknowledgements   *144*

# Introduction

Few areas of women's health stir up as much confusion and debate as hormone replacement therapy or HRT, which arouses both condemnation and enthusiasm in equal measure.

The vast majority of women who are likely candidates for HRT are at a time in their lives when their hormones are in decline – between the ages of 50 and 60. What could be more natural than to 'pop-a-pill' to alleviate their menopausal symptoms, rejuvenate their middle years, and ensure a healthy old age? For there has been such an improvement in the quality of women's lives that the proportion of women living past the age of menopause has tripled during the past century, and is expected to increase steadily in the foreseeable future.

If adulthood is defined as beginning at the age of 21, the average age at natural menopause is 51 and the average life expectancy is 81, then women in the United States, in Europe, and in much of the developed world will live one-half of their lives in the years after menopause, a time of relative oestrogen deficiency compared to their reproductive years.

The impact of this deficiency on some of our lives is so dramatic that we look for a medication to relieve its symptoms, and hormone replacement therapy may well be suggested by our doctors.

It should be a straightforward decision. But our hormonal patterns are as individual to us as our fingerprints, and it is not possible that the same hormonal preparation will suit every woman. Not only that, but for all its possible benefits, HRT carries potential risks.

Is it really possible for doctors to enhance a woman's quality of life by prescribing a medication and also to tell them this medication has some risks outweighing the benefits?

The confusion is fuelled by the media when it reports the latest research into some aspect of HRT which appears to contradict previous findings. Furthermore, few doctors suggest natural alternatives to their patients: while some such natural remedies make dubious claims, others have gained a respectable track record of efficacy, and are available from pharmacies, an increasing number of health food outlets and company websites.

This book sets out to present the facts and fiction about both hormone replacement therapy and its natural alternatives. Threading through the chapters are 'personal profiles' of women who have written to me about their experiences of both. Once you have read the book, you will be able to create your own 'personal profile' and thus make an informed choice about a decision that could affect the rest of your life.

I hope you will share this book with someone close to you.

Headaches, depression and anxiety can be unsettling during your menopausal transition.

# 1

# Hormonal highways

# Hormones and your body

Perhaps you have picked up this book because your doctor has recommended hormone replacement therapy for your menopausal symptoms, saying that the hot flushes and dreadful night sweats which have troubled you for the past few weeks will vanish. What a relief that would be! Nevertheless, you have decided to find out more about it before committing yourself.

Or maybe you are shortly to undergo a hysterectomy, and the consultant wants to remove your ovaries at the same time. The doctors say they serve no useful purpose now that you are menopausal, and the words 'ovarian cancer' have been mentioned. As you have completed your family, you are quite happy to follow this advice. In passing, your consultant has mentioned that you should take HRT after the operation. This has alarmed you because your sister takes it and has gained a huge amount of weight – you wonder if this will happen to you.

Or perhaps you found yourself bursting into tears one day at work when your boss commented on your lack of concentration. It's true that your memory has not been as razor-sharp as usual. As you later told the doctor, you are also sleeping fitfully and have gone right off sex. Your doctor thinks your symptoms indicate the menopause, and recommends HRT as the solution to them. But you do not want to take it – you are sure there are other, perhaps more natural, ways to deal with your present situation.

Or possibly you are a young woman whose whole life is ruled by the agony of endometriosis, and every conventional drug available has failed to provide long-term sustainable relief. Surgery is now the only option, but this will entail removal of your ovaries, and means you will never have children. You are likely to experience your menopause within two years. The consultant has recommended HRT after surgery as the only way to alleviate the symptoms. You are baffled about this as it means replacing your own hormones with manufactured ones, so you have resolved to find out more about HRT.

Or you are in your late 60s and, while attending a cardiac rehabilitation unit at hospital following a heart attack, have agreed to take part in a clinical trial of low-dosage HRT. The improvement in your life has been dramatic – you feel more energetic and lively than you have done for years, and sexual intimacy has again become pleasurable now that your vagina is moist and soft. But a nagging anxiety disturbs your happy frame of mind – your mother died of uterine cancer when she was 75, and you want to know more about the risks for you if you continue with HRT.

You may have been surprised to read the scenarios above, having thought that HRT is relevant only when a woman is in her 50s and menopausal. What they reflect is how our lives are continually influenced by our own particular 'hormonal highways' – at different stages of our lives, the influences of different hormones become more prominent according to changing circumstances.

Taking time to pause and reflect on changes in your emotional and physical life can be very helpful.

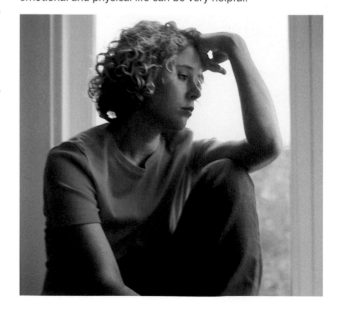

# The endocrine system

Hormonal highways develop through the endocrine system – a number of glands that produce hormones. Endocrine glands work as a team and include the following:

- **The pituitary** Located at the base of the brain, the pituitary is responsible for the secretion of two hormones essential to the reproductive system: follicle-stimulating hormone (FSH) and luteinizing hormone (LH). Its main activity is the control of the other endocrine glands.

- **The thyroid** Consisting of two lobes, one either side of the trachea (windpipe), the thyroid produces two hormones essential for normal metabolic processes and mental and physical development: T3 and thyroxine, or T4. T3 has a role in influencing mood and emotion, but its primary role is an accelerator of metabolism in all organs of the body.

- **The parathyroids** Usually four in number and found on the back and side of each thyroid lobe, the parathyroids produce hormones that increase the amount of calcium circulating in the blood.

- **The adrenals** These consist of a flattened body above each kidney and are made up of a cortex and a medulla. The adrenal cortex produces several hormones including cortisol (which is important in carbohydrate breakdown and in the normal response to stress) and the sex hormones (oestrogens and androgens). In men, androgens have an important role in stimulating the development of the sex organs and the principal source of these hormones is the testes. However, androgen hormones produced by the adrenals also have a vital role in women. After the

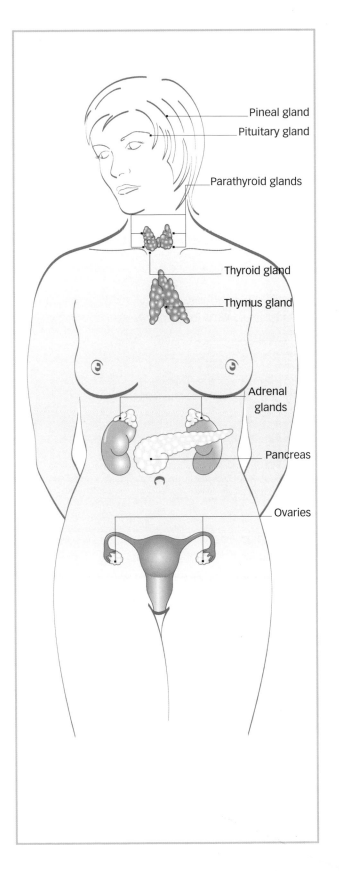

Pineal gland
Pituitary gland
Parathyroid glands
Thyroid gland
Thymus gland
Adrenal glands
Pancreas
Ovaries

menopause, some androgens, such as dehydroepiandrosterone (DHEA) and androstenedione, can be converted by the adrenals into oestrone, a weak oestrogen. This becomes the body's main source of oestrogen when the ovaries have stopped producing it. The adrenal medulla secretes adrenaline (epinephrine) involved in the 'flight or fight' response when in danger or under emotional or physical stress. A slow, rather irregular release of adrenaline goes on all the time, but a real boost to production is any situation fraught with fear or anger. When that happens, adrenaline increases the blood flow to the muscles by accelerating the heart rate and shutting off the less essential blood flow to skin and intestines.

- **The pancreas** This gland, which is located near the stomach, produces insulin, the hormone that regulates the level of sugar in the blood. Insulin works by making it easier for glucose to enter the cells, where it is used as fuel.

- **The ovaries** In addition to producing eggs, the ovaries produce the hormones oestrogen and progesterone (in response to FSH and LH from the pituitary gland) and testosterone.

## What are hormones?

The word hormone comes from a Greek word horman, meaning 'to stir up or arouse to activity', and this is exactly what hormones do. These chemical substances are made in minute quantities in glands, and circulate around the body via the bloodstream. Each one has a specific effect on its target organ or tissue, controlling, activating and directing structures and functions. Many hormones affect the urges, desires and feelings which are yours and nobody elses. Fluctuating hormone levels will vary throughout your life, influencing your moods, activities and sensitivities as they ebb and flow.

**Hormones also:**
- affect metabolic rate (how quickly/slowly you function)
- trigger growth (as at puberty – from about nine years old)
- balance blood sugar
- affect the body's water balance
- regulate respiration (your breathing)
- determine cell metabolism (the rate at which cells function)
- affect neural activity (your nervous system).

So you can see what a varied and complex part hormones play in your life and how much they matter. One hormone cannot be viewed in isolation but must be seen in its physiological context as a component in the whole balance of circulating hormones.

## A question of balance

Some women live their whole lives with no hormonal problems whatsoever. Periods come and go with minimum disruption, pre-menstrual syndrome (PMS) is unknown, there is little or no trouble before and after pregnancy – even the contraceptive pill is swallowed without side-effects – and sterilization or hysterectomy produce no more than transitory difficulties.

But for other women, any interference with the hormonal system at any level causes chemical changes and alterations in body/mind rhythms with resulting symptoms of hormonal distress.

**Hormonal upset can arise from:**
- the use of the birth control pill or other hormone-containing medicines
- hypothalamic or pituitary problems resulting from pregnancy, miscarriage or abortion
- surgery such as tubal ligation (sterilization) or hysterectomy

- anorexia or bulimia
- trauma (e.g. as a victim of violence)
- conditions such as ovarian cysts, polycystic ovaries, endometriosis or uterine fibroids.

Changes in hormone levels can also occur if the immune system breaks down as a result of chemical poisoning or viral infection, for hormonal problems and immune system dysfunction are often linked. For example, the main problem may be hormonal imbalance, but this is exacerbated by an impaired immune system function causing chronic tiredness. Or the basic problem may be centred on the immune system, causing damage to the ovaries and thus affecting hormonal status.

Stress and lifestyle will always play their part. For instance, female airline flight attendants frequently suffer menstrual instability because their biological 'time clocks' are disrupted as they fly through different time zones. Similarly, dancers, who need lean, muscular bodies, often experience amenorrhoea (an abnormal suppression or absence of menstruation). Traumatic experiences such as bereavement, divorce and violence all destabilize hormonal equilibrium, as can redundancy and moving home.

**Ovarian cysts** An ovarian cyst is an abnormal, fluid-filled swelling that develops in the ovary. The most common type occurs when the egg-producing follicle of the ovary enlarges to produce a 'follicular cyst'. Cysts often produce no symptoms but some cause acute pain or irregular bleeding.

**Polycystic ovaries** This condition is thought to occur due to an imbalance between luteinizing hormone and follicle-stimulating hormone, produced by the pituitary gland. Multiple cysts develop in either one or both ovaries and ovulation ceases.

**Endometriosis** This is a condition in which the cells that form the endometrium (lining of the uterus) develop outside their normal location, forming little clusters of tissue (called implants) outside the uterus.

**Fibroids** These are lumps of fibrous and muscular tissue found growing on all levels of the uterus, although they have also been discovered in other areas within the pelvis. They are known to shrink naturally in women as they near the menopause, but some researchers believe they are sensitive to oestrogen and are more likely to grow when high levels of this hormone are present.

Frequent flying between different time zones can disrupt your biological 'time clock'.

# The ovarian hormones

Of especial importance to women are the three hormones produced by the ovaries: oestrogen, progesterone and testosterone.

## OESTROGEN

Oestrogen is not really a single hormone: the word refers to a class of hormones that control female sexual development and promote the growth and function of female sex organs and secondary sexual characteristics. These oestrogens include the hormones oestradiol and oestrone, which are essential for the health of the reproductive organs, and oestriol, the predominant oestrogen hormone during pregnancy.

Your body began producing oestrogen when you were no more than a foetus, 15–20 weeks old, in your mother's womb. No doubt you have marvelled at the exquisitely soft skin of a baby – this is due to oestrogen, which causes an extra layer of fat to develop and so makes the skin ultra soft.

At puberty, your level of oestrogen increased dramatically, albeit erratically: your breasts developed and the distribution of your body fat changed to produce the rounded contours of feminine hips and thighs – this is often described as 'puppy fat'. Maybe you can remember some of your emotions during puberty and adolescence – one day feeling elated and raring to go, the next apathetic and unhappy. These fluctuations are hardly surprising, given the bewildering and intricate changes that occur as your hormonal balance is established.

From this time your life became influenced by the cyclic monthly changes involved in menstruation as hormone levels rise and fall. For example, you may feel the stirrings of desire and the onset of sexual hunger in mid-cycle, at about the time your basal temperature readings indicate that you are at or near ovulation. This is the time at which

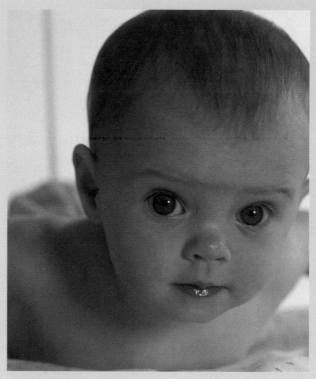

You can see how this baby's skin is beautifully soft and unblemished because of oestrogen.

both oestrogen and progesterone levels peak, indicating a readiness for pregnancy.

Oestrogen contributes to a healthy sex life, causing the vagina to moisten when aroused, and sensual areas to respond to stimulation.

As levels of oestrogen decline during the menopausal years, the vaginal tissues become thinner and dryer. Oestrogenic lubrication for sexual activity diminishes, and can result in vaginal penetration becoming uncomfortable and painful.

## PROGESTERONE

Progesterone is produced primarily by the ovaries, although smaller amounts are also produced by the adrenal glands and large amounts by the placenta during pregnancy. Its role is to maintain the healthy functioning of the female reproductive system.

At the time of ovulation, the ovaries dramatically increase their output of progesterone, stimulating a woman's sex drive and preparing the lining of the uterus for fertilization. Adequate levels of progesterone are essential to the survival of the fertilized egg and the foetus. They are also thought to be responsible for the sense of well-being that is experienced by some women during their pregnancies.

Progesterone is known to be linked with mood and emotion. If you feel under par or even suffer pre-menstrual syndrome (PMS) at certain stages of your menstrual cycle, it may be likely to be due to low levels of the hormone progesterone.

It was the pioneering British gynaecologist, Dr Katherina Dalton, who pioneered the addition of progesterone for sufferers of PMS. She used to experience terrible migraines with her menstrual cycle and discovered these could be alleviated by progesterone injections. What led her to this discovery was the realization that her migraines completely disappeared during the final months of her pregnancy, which is when progesterone levels in the body soar. However, not all women in this situation respond in the way she did.

Apart from its reproductive function, progesterone is needed for the production of other hormones such as cortisol, which has an important role in the metabolism of carbohydrates, fats and proteins, and in the body's response to injury and infection.

The production of ovarian progesterone declines during the menopausal years as the reproductive process ends. But it is still very much involved throughout your body, as explained on page 62.

Hormonal balance contributes to the glow of healthy happiness seen in a pregnant woman.

## PROGESTERONE CREAM
Nowadays, the most successful and most widely used type of progesterone preparation is transdermal progesterone (see page 65). This comes in the form of a cream and is applied to the skin. The progesterone is absorbed rapidly.

## TESTOSTERONE

As well as being a major hormone for men, testosterone is also of great importance for women. Not only are the levels of testosterone in women's blood higher than the levels of oestrogen, but their brains contain 20 times more testosterone than oestrogen.

Men have 10–20 times more free testosterone than women – one-half of a woman's testosterone is produced in the ovary and the other half in the adrenal gland. The hormone helps to determine secondary sexual characteristics such as muscle mass and patterns of hair growth, and adequate levels are essential for sexual desire, activity and responsiveness in both men and women.

Nevertheless, while testosterone fuels the flames of desire, psychological factors determine the intensity and direction of the flame. The commonly held belief that hormones, in general, are the primary motivators of sexual activity in humans is a gross over-simplification: hormones do not cause behaviour, rather they raise the likelihood that a given behaviour will occur. Habit, circumstance, expectation and conditioning can all have a more profound effect on behaviour than hormones.

Testosterone levels reduce by about one-third in the average post-menopausal woman who still has her ovaries. If her ovaries are removed, the fall of testosterone is twice as great.

Hypothalamus releasing hormones

Pituitary gland

Ovary

Corpus luteum

Breast

Follicle

Womb lining

Fallopian tube

Ovary

Early embryo

Vagina

➤ Progesterone

➤ Oestrogen

➤ Luteinizing hormone

➤ Follicle-stimulating hormone

## THE HORMONE LOOP

Throughout the month, a constant feedback loop creates a continuous adjustment and regulation of the hormone levels between the hypothalamus and pituitary, and the ovaries.

# The change

The three hormones described on the preceding pages – oestrogen, progesterone and testosterone – constantly change from day to day in a predictable and orderly rhythm. They are key to the time spanning the years during which a woman is at her reproductive prime. This is a process with a beginning, a peak, a decline and an end – and, interestingly, humans are the only mammals in the world to experience this, all other female mammals reproduce until they die.

Central to a woman's reproductive life are her two ovaries. Estimates vary, but it is believed there are 6–7 million eggs present in a female foetus by the middle of its gestation. These begin to die off even before the child is born, but even so, the ovaries at birth contain somewhere between half-a-million and five million eggs. As the child develops the eggs continue to die off, so that by the time she reaches puberty, there are between 200,000 and 300,000 eggs.

During a woman's fertile years, one of her ovaries will ripen and release an egg once a month.

**Peri-menopause** This is the period approximately two years before and two years after your final menstrual period. This is the time when you will notice the most physical changes, such as irregular periods and hot flushes, for example.

**Menopause** Your final menstrual period. Determining the date of your menopause can only be done retrospectively after you have been free of menstruation for a full year.

**Post-menopause** These are the months and years that follow your final menstrual period. It overlaps with the peri-menopausal stage.

**Climacteric** The term 'climacteric' comes from a Greek word meaning 'rung of a ladder' and refers to the period of passage out of the reproductive stage of your life and into the non-reproductive phase. It encompasses peri-menopause, menopause and the early post-menopausal years.

Each time a woman ovulates, not one or two, but between 20 and 1,000 eggs are used up. Only one or two eggs per cycle would have fully matured, and with increasing age, the eggs become used up more rapidly. Between the ages of 38 and 44, about 50,000 eggs are lost.

Ovulation slows down during the peri-menopause: this is defined as the transition between the time you begin to experience menopausal symptoms (usually the mid to late 40s) and the time when your periods actually stop (average age of 51).

Many women find that they experience the menopause at the same age as their mothers did.

## How do I know if I'm in my peri-menopause?

The signs that herald the arrival of the peri-menopause are varied. You might find yourself having two periods a month, and if you get a heavier flow, you may think you are always bleeding. Or you could go several months without bleeding. The actual flow may change, with lighter, more watery bleeding and less clotting due to reduced oestrogen levels. The wide-ranging hormone-related symptoms of the peri-menopause can be bothersome and include:

- night sweats, interrupted sleep or insomnia
- irritability
- anxiety
- loss of concentration
- headaches (especially pre-menstrual migraines)
- vaginal dryness
- vaginal atrophy (thinning of the vaginal walls due to lack of oestrogen)
- less interest in sex
- urinary stress incontinence
- mood swings.

Obviously, many of these symptoms are interconnected. For instance, if you have such severe night sweats that you develop insomnia, your concentration will suffer and you will be irritable.

## Reverse puberty

Any mood swings may well strike a chord with your early adolescence, and indeed these hormonal changes are just like those at puberty. As mentioned earlier, an erratic production of oestrogen played an essential part in your development at puberty. The fluctuating hormonal levels, coupled with the daily traumas of adolescent life, lead to the wild mood swings that are so much a part of being a pubescent girl.

In the peri-menopause, the exact reverse happens but with similar results: the ovaries are winding down instead of gearing up, but the duelling hormonal levels can bring on the same mood swings you probably experienced all those years ago.

## Is it me – or is it hot today?

The most commonly experienced peri-menopausal symptoms are hot flushes and night sweats. These occur in up to 25 per cent of peri-menopausal women and 50–85 per cent of menopausal women experience them. For most women, they happen over a period of one to two years, but in 20–25 per cent they continue for more than five years.

Hot flushes can cause considerable surprise and embarrassment. One day you are busy in the office as usual, the next moment you suddenly feel a warm sensation rising up from your chest, spreading across your neck, up to your head and scalp... it's boiling hot in the room, beads of perspiration prickle your skin. After what seems an age, the heat is gone, you are wet with sweat and almost immediately you begin to feel chilled.

**The sudden onset of a hot flush can be very unsettling, a feeling that continues until it has passed.**

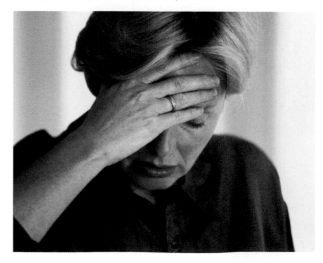

A typical hot flush lasts no more than three minutes, but it can range in duration from a few seconds to half-an-hour. It can be experienced in different ways. Some women have a specific focal point, such as the skin between the breasts, where the first tingles are felt, warning of an approaching hot flush. There may be no outward sign of redness or sweating – or you might sweat profusely and become as red as a beetroot. The degree of sensation varies from mild discomfort to such intense feelings that you have to fight the urge to pull off your clothing.

At night, the flushes are called night sweats, and you may wake up to find yourself drenched in sweat, and need to dry yourself and change your night clothes. Women often complain that night sweats are worse than daytime flushes because:

- it is not possible to pick up the warning signals of an approaching flush while asleep, and do anything to lessen its impact
- disturbed sleep results in tiredness, depression and irritability next day.

## WHY DO HOT FLUSHES HAPPEN?

The physiology of hot flushes is not yet fully understood, but they are due to chemicals being released into the bloodstream at this time of hormonal disruption. The blood vessels are sensitive to the chemicals and dilate, so blood rushes to the skin, making you hot and red. A medical dictionary defines hot flushes as 'vasomotor symptoms of the climacterium – sudden vasodilation with a sensation of heat, usually involving the face and neck, and upper part of the chest; sweats, often profuse, frequently follow the flush'.

Hot flushes are termed 'vasomotor' symptoms because the size of the blood vessels changes as part of the body's temperature-control system – blood vessels dilate (get larger) to allow more blood through so that you can cool down. They are linked to the breakdown of

> **DID YOU KNOW?**
> Not all oestrogen is lost when ovarian function ceases. The conversion of adrenal-gland hormones into oestrogen (which had little importance before menopause) increases. This oestrogen conversion occurs primarily in fat tissues. Because of this process, oestrogen production continues for at least 10-20 years after menopause. This can be quite variable from woman to woman, which helps to explain why some women age more rapidly than others (an acceleration of skin ageing is likely as oestrogen levels decline).

temperature control by the hypothalamus as oestrogen production declines. Hot flushes signal the completion of your life as a potential bearer of children for, at or near your menopause:

- your ovaries have used up all their eggs
- they therefore no longer respond to the secretion of FSH from the pituitary as they once did by producing oestrogen.

A few women go through the peri-menopause overnight – periods will simply cease and these women have no associated symptoms. But most women experience some discomfort at this time and are aware of hormonal changes going on within their bodies which may or may not disrupt their lives. This is usually an erratic process: periods may come late or early, may be short or long, light or heavy – or vanish for months and then suddenly reappear. It can take between two and five years to complete and enormous changes take place in a woman's body as it acquires a new balance with lower levels of hormones.

The menopause is considered complete when periods have not occurred for one whole year.

# Surgical removal of ovaries

For some women the removal of the ovaries may be the only option if severe symptoms of pain, PMS or endometriosis (see page 13) persist and all other treatments have been tried or if the ovaries are diseased.

Endometriosis is a disease affecting many women in their reproductive years and it will recur while there is ovarian function. Although the ovaries themselves may be healthy, surgery involving hysterectomy and removal of the ovaries is the only permanent cure. Endometriosis is the only disease that is 'treated' by the surgical removal of tissue not directly affected by the disorder.

Some doctors advise against hormone replacement therapy for the first six months after surgery to remove ovaries. If all the endometrial implants are removed during the operation, then the chance of a recurrence of the disease is slim – however, if even the tiniest deposit remains, then HRT will assist its growth.

All too often removal of ovaries is recommended for women aged 50+ who are having a hysterectomy, on the grounds that ovarian cancer may develop if they are retained. There is still considerable controversy about this issue, and if you are faced with this possibility, you need to weigh the risks of developing ovarian cancer against the benefits of continued ovarian function (i.e. hormone production). The latest research in the USA, Denmark, Japan and Australia, as well as that undertaken by Cancer Research in the UK, indicates the following:

- Family risk factors include infertility, a well-documented family history of ovarian cancer, late menopause and lack of child-bearing.
- Sterilization may reduce the risk of ovarian cancer by 39 per cent.
- Hysterectomy may reduce the risk of ovarian cancer by 36 per cent (although the Danish nationwide controlled follow-up study of ovarian cancer after hysterectomy (1997) suggests this protection might fade out with time).
- Women preserving at least one ovary have a significantly decreased risk of ovarian cancer for at least ten years after hysterectomy.
- Women who had heavy periods before hysterectomy tended to have a lower risk of ovarian cancer after surgery than women who had light or normal periods.

If you are still ovulating, then removing your ovaries will deprive you of significant hormonal support which is difficult to replace adequately. The most critical issue is loss of bone mass leading to osteoporosis, which surgical removal of ovaries is known to initiate (see page 44). In menopausal years the ovaries continue to secrete hormones which will support your well-being and health.

## PREMATURE MENOPAUSE

Whether you are 20 or 50 years old, surgical removal of ovaries is a very serious step to take (see also page 61). It leads to a premature menopause either straightaway or within two years of the operation, and you are likely to be prescribed HRT. This may result in months of trial and error until the correct dosage is found to supplement your own reduced oestrogen levels.

## IMPORTANT

It is vitally important that you discuss all the issues and implications of HRT with your doctor if your ovaries are to be surgically removed.

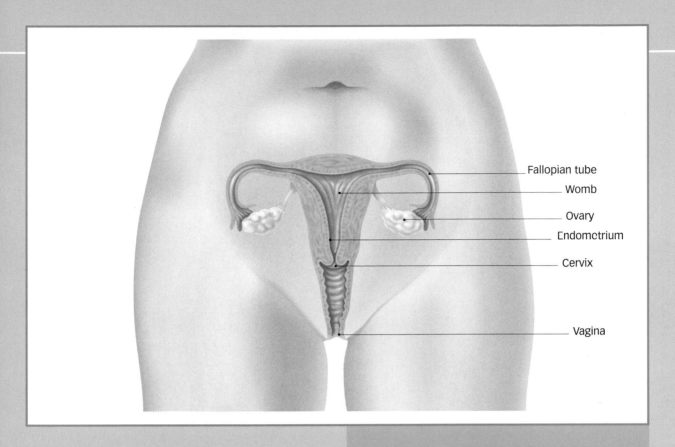

Fallopian tube

Womb

Ovary

Endometrium

Cervix

Vagina

## THE REPRODUCTIVE SYSTEM

The main components of the reproductive system are the womb (uterus), Fallopian tubes and ovaries. The outlet of the womb is the cervix which projects into the vagina.

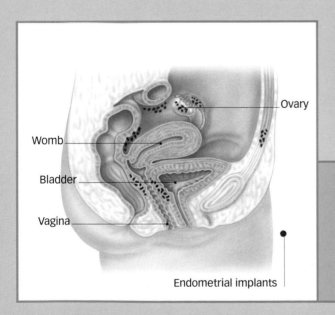

Ovary

Womb

Bladder

Vagina

Endometrial implants

## ENDOMETRIOSIS

Here are some of the internal organs where deposits of endometriosis are commonly found.

2

# Hormone replacement therapy

# Considering hormone replacement therapy

Ever since the hormone oestrogen was first found to be linked with the menopause, early in the twentieth century, attempts have been made to use it as a medication to alleviate menopausal symptoms. In the 1920s, extracts from the dried ovaries of sheep were used in early trials, and in the 1930s a 'natural oestrogen' extracted from the urine of pregnant mares was found to be effective.

By the mid-1960s oestrogen therapy was hailed as 'the pathway to eternal youth', promising to protect women from the 'living decay' of their middle years. Wrinkly skin, middle-age spread and sagging breasts would be eradicated along with crying spells, violent mood swings, aching joints and loss of memory. Replacing all this would be eternally feminine, sexually active menopausal women with glowing skin and glossy hair.

A driving force in the promotion of oestrogen therapy at this time was a New York gynaecologist, Dr Robert Wilson, founder of the Wilson Foundation. The pharmaceutical industry generously contributed millions of dollars to the Foundation and funded aggressive promotional and advertising campaigns. Dr Wilson's book, *Feminine Forever*, sold over 100,000 copies in its first year. Women's magazines eagerly seized upon his ideas, spreading the belief that the menopause was a kind of 'living decay'.

By feeding on women's greatest fears, Dr Wilson struck a receptive chord. He extolled the virtues of oestrogen replacement, which would save women from 'the tragedy of menopause which often destroys their character as

well as their health'. Fuelled by a potent cocktail of vanity, anxiety and media coverage, sales of oestrogen rocketed – even though there had been no formal assessment as to its safety, let alone its long-term effects.

In the 1970s, however, panic set in when medical research showed that American women who took oestrogen were 5–14 times more likely to develop cancer of the lining of the uterus (the endometrium) than those who were not taking oestrogen. It appeared that the hormone stimulated growth of the endometrium and that this was leading to cancer in some cases. Understandably, the popularity of oestrogen therapy waned.

New approaches were needed. One was the addition of progestogen (a synthetic form of the hormone progesterone) to the therapeutic regime. This 'opposes' the action of the oestrogen and allows the lining of the womb to be shed, as in a normal period, thus reducing the risk of cancer developing.

At this point the pharmaceutical industry abandoned its false claims that oestrogen therapy preserved feminine

Lines and wrinkles are not something to be ashamed of – laughter lines reflect a contented life in middle years.

beauty and started to proclaim that the primary objective of the new 'hormone replacement therapy' was the relief of menopausal symptoms.

## So what exactly is HRT?

Hormone replacement therapy is an available treatment to replace, or top-up, a woman's oestrogen levels when levels produced by the ovaries decrease during the menopause. As mentioned earlier, oestrogen on its own provides no protection against the possibility of uterine cancer, and you will need this unless you have had a hysterectomy. The addition of a synthetic hormone, progestogen, provides that protection since it is not chemically possible to manufacture natural progesterone.

Although progestogens are able to fulfil many of the functions of progesterone, the human body has a certain degree of difficulty 'recognizing' and coping with them. This is the cause of the well-known side-effects of mood swings and depression, which some women have when they start HRT.

The oestrogen used in HRT comes in two basic forms: 'synthetic' (produced in a laboratory from soy beans) and 'natural' (extracted from pigs' ovaries or the urine of pregnant mares). The latter is used in the manufacture of two commonly prescribed preparations called Premarin and Prempak C. If you are concerned about animal welfare, you may not be too happy about taking an HRT preparation produced in this way.

In many ways the hormones used in HRT are exactly the same as the ones used in the contraceptive pill. The differences lies in the source of the oestrogen and the dose – HRT uses either synthetic oestrogen or 'natural' oestrogen extracted from pigs' ovaries or pregnant mares' urine, whereas the contraceptive pill contains the synthetic form of oestrogen called ethinyl oestradiol. The dose of oestrogen is also much lower in HRT preparations.

The progestogens used in the contraceptive pill and HRT are the same, the difference lies in the schedule – in HRT they are given for only 10–12 days of each menstrual cycle.

## Why should I consider taking HRT?

First, HRT is one option for you if symptoms of your climacteric are disrupting your physical and emotional well-being. You can assess the severity or otherwise of these by completing the chart on page 26.

Secondly, HRT can provide protection from the possibility of either cardiovascular disease or osteoporosis as you age, particularly if you are at risk from either condition for genetic or other reasons. In recent years, promising evidence has also emerged that it may offer protection against Alzheimer's disease (see pages 41–42) and bowel cancer (see pages 42–43).

### DID YOU KNOW?

For six months of their pregnancies, an estimated 75,000 mares are confined in stalls on farms in Canada and the USA. These stalls are so small that the mares are unable to take a step or two in any direction. A harness is tied to the animal's rear quarters from which is attached a cumbersome urine-collection bag. This chafes their legs and prevents them from lying down comfortably. Outside exercise is occasional, if at all, and mares are given limited drinking water so that their urine will yield more concentrated oestrogens. Some of the foals born are used to replace their exhausted mothers, many of whom have been confined on these farms for up to 20 years. But most are sold, fattened and slaughtered for pet food.

## MENOPAUSAL SYMPTOM CHART

*Tick the box that most closely reflects how severely you are experiencing each of these symptoms. Each box you ticked has a score beside it.*

| Symptoms | Severe | Moderate | Mild | None |
|---|---|---|---|---|
| Hot flushes | 12☐ | 8☐ | 4☐ | 0☐ |
| Sweating attacks | 12☐ | 8☐ | 4☐ | 0☐ |
| Tension/irritability | 3☐ | 2☐ | 1☐ | 0☐ |
| Dryness of vagina/irritation | 3☐ | 2☐ | 1☐ | 0☐ |
| Loss of interest in sexual intimacy (ignore if not applicable) | 3☐ | 2☐ | 1☐ | 0☐ |
| Insomnia | 3☐ | 2☐ | 1☐ | 0☐ |
| Lack of energy | 3☐ | 2☐ | 1☐ | 0☐ |
| Hair/skin changes | 3☐ | 2☐ | 1☐ | 0☐ |
| Muscular and/or joint pains | 3☐ | 2☐ | 1☐ | 0☐ |
| Changes in memory/concentration | 3☐ | 2☐ | 1☐ | 0☐ |

*Once you have ticked a box for each symptom, add up your score. A score of 30 or more strongly suggests that symptoms are associated with the menopause, although a low score will not exclude this.*

# Will the doctor do any tests before prescribing it?

Your doctor should examine you thoroughly, especially your breasts and pelvis, and check your blood pressure. There are a few medical reasons for not giving HRT and it may not be suitable if you have a history of any of the following conditions:

- Endometriosis (unless it has been treated or has become quiescent post-menopausally)
- Breast cancer or cysts
- Cancer of the lining of the womb (the endometrium)
- Liver disease
- High blood pressure or if you have had a stroke
- A personal and/or family history of clotting of the deep leg veins or the lungs
- Any oestrogen-dependent malignancy
- Untreated vaginal bleeding.

It is unlikely that you will be required to take a blood test, even though some of us manufacture more oestrogen in our bodies than others, so the dose regimens for HRT should be individualized according to our hormone levels. For the most part, blood tests to accurately measure the levels of hormones in your body are useless and extremely unreliable.

The tests are only able to measure 1–9 per cent of the biologically active hormones circulating in your body. There is now a better way. The World Health Organization for the last five years has been using saliva samples for an accurate reading of hormone levels.

When your saliva gland makes saliva it also secretes the biologically active forms of cortisone, testosterone, oestrogen and progesterone. This makes it possible to measure the levels of these hormones in a saliva test.

Your blood pressure should be monitored regularly by your doctor if you take HRT.

The Female Hormone Kit test, for example, is a very simple one which can be done in the privacy of your home with the samples you collect being sent for analysis. A total of 11 saliva samples are collected at specific times, and levels of oestrogen, progesterone and testosterone are mapped to provide an accurate picture of your 'hormonal highways'. An interpretation of the test is provided when the results are returned. If you decide to have this test, you could discuss the findings with your doctor during the initial discussion about taking HRT.

> *I had awful night sweats and within days of going on HRT I felt a different person. I had so much more energy. I hadn't realized I was lacking it as I think it tends to build up gradually and you get used to it.*
>
> *It's also helped me cope with work and my family better, especially as my husband and I are now managing a country hotel – I'm sure I couldn't work such long hours without HRT.*
>
> **LYNN (Wales)**

# Benefits and side-effects

## What are the benefits if I take HRT for menopausal symptoms?

As soon as you start taking HRT you are likely to find an improvement in the frequency and severity of hot flushes and night sweats, maybe within a week. This often has a 'knock-on' effect in that your sleeping patterns will improve which in turn will reduce any daytime irritability, mood swings, etc. Women often report a general improvement in their energy levels, their ability to cope with the unexpected and in their overall outlook and self-confidence. The full effect should be apparent by 12 weeks, when you should have your first critical review.

Relief from menopausal symptoms can transform your life.

### IS HRT THE ANSWER TO ALL SYMPTOMS?
HRT can be a useful diagnostic tool in eliminating symptoms which are oestrogen-dependent. For instance, you might find that HRT has abolished your mood swings and irritability, yet you remain significantly depressed. If that happens, additional help, such as counselling, might be suggested by your doctor.

## What about side-effects?

HRT causes 'start-up' effects. These are the consequence of your body reacting to the presence once again of normal, adult levels of oestradiol in your blood, sometimes after an absence of many years. You are highly likely to experience some, or all, of the following:

- Breast tenderness
- Nipple sensitivity
- Headaches
- Increase in appetite
- Calf muscle cramps.

Infrequent or rare reactions include:

- Diarrhoea
- Gastro-intestinal upsets
- Muscular or joint pains
- Scalp hair loss
- Increased blood pressure
- Sensitivity to light
- Vaginal bleeding
- Breathing disorders
- Depression
- Acne
- Pains or swelling in upper leg
- Skin rash
- Heart palpitations
- Swollen ankles
- Migraines.

If you experience any of these, you should see your doctor and discuss the situation, rather than waiting for your first critical review at the end of 12 weeks.

# HRT and weight gain

You may have friends or family who have gained weight when taking HRT, and this could be one of your greatest concerns – will it happen to me?

In midlife, women tend to gain weight whether menopausal or not. However, after the menopause, this extra weight is distributed more in the abdomen than in the thighs and hips. Hormone replacement therapy effectively prevents the redistribution of body fat, but does not prevent the weight gain itself.

Logic dictates that a gain in weight is inevitable if you take oestrogen, for this turns the food energy into body fat – it is no coincidence that cattle are fed on this hormone to fatten them up for market. A 'sudden' increase in weight is a common complaint after starting HRT, and the reason weight-gain continues to rise is likely to be a combination of HRT, overeating and inadequate physical exercise.

Research has shown that women on HRT do gain weight, reality tells a different story, as borne out by anecdotal evidence.

If weight gain is an issue for you, prepare a diet diary if you are considering HRT or are on HRT. Take a separate page for each day of the week and on each one, line up columns with the following headings:

- Time you ate
- What food you consumed
- How much you ate
- What you were doing when you ate
- Where you ate
- With whom you ate, or if alone
- How you felt when you ate.

Keeping this record will make you far more aware of what you really eat, and the psychological stimuli associated with your food intake. You might be surprised by what is revealed. For example, many people find that they 'snack' much more than they realized, or that they eat more if they are alone.

Make a note of your weight on day 1 of starting HRT, record your diet diary (honestly!) for two weeks, and if you have put on weight, take immediate action. Discontinue the HRT for two weeks and monitor your weight. If it stays the same, moderate and/or modify your food intake, and increase your physical exercise. Then continue the HRT for two weeks and moderate and/or modify your food intake, as well as increasing your physical exercise.

If you continue to gain weight in spite of making lifestyle changes, then you may need to discontinue the HRT and seek other solutions for your menopausal difficulties.

> *I had a hysterectomy and oophorectomy when I was 30 years old because of phase 4 endometriosis. Severe hot flushes and sweats started during the first two to four weeks after surgery and I gained about 60-70lb (27–32 kilos) during the year I was on HRT. At first I used patches but the glue caused a severe rash, so I went on to Premarin (oestrogen-only tablets). I decided to stop taking it and see how I felt. After several months I went to the doctor and told him my menopausal symptoms had gone, so he agreed it was alright not to take HRT but that I would need regular bone scans.*
>
> *I lost about 20lb (9 kilos) in weight after stopping HRT and checking into a healthier eating lifestyle – I don't agree with so much emphasis on raw foods, but I now eat more fruit and vegetables and have cut down on salt and fried foods.*
>
> **STEPHANIE (Wales)**

# What types of HRT are available?

HRT preparations come in various different forms. The main choices on offer at the present time, all of which contain various dosages of hormones, are tablets, patches, implants, nasal sprays, vaginal creams and rings.

## TABLETS

This is the most common form of HRT and there are more than 50 different tablets available. For women who have not had a hysterectomy (i.e. who have an intact uterus), tablets containing both oestrogen and progestogen are prescribed. Sometimes the two hormones are combined in one tablet, sometimes they are taken separately in one of the following ways:

- **Cyclical therapy** Oestrogen is taken for the first 21 days of the cycle; progestogen is taken from day 9 to day 21. Thus from day 21 there are seven days with no medication. Two days after the tablets are stopped, the fall in artificial hormone levels induces the lining of the womb to be shed, resulting in withdrawal bleeding. Such bleeds are not true periods, but should resemble them in being of less than a week's duration, not unduly heavy, relatively pain-free and on time.
- **Continuous therapy** Oestrogen is taken continuously every day and progestogen is taken from day 14 to day 25 of the menstrual cycle. Once the progestogen is finished, a withdrawal bleed is induced in the same way as in cyclical therapy. Continuous therapy is only prescribed for women over 54 years old or who have been without a period for one year.

### Advantages of tablets
- Convenience – they are neat and easy to pack when travelling and it is simple to 'pop-a-pill'.
- It is easy to alter the dosage level if necessary.

### Disadvantages of tablets
- Irritation of a monthly bleed, especially if you thought your menopause meant freedom from menstruation.
- Some spotting and occasional bleeding is not unusual in the first six months of continuous therapy, and many women therefore prefer the predictability of the cyclic method. However, if you are willing to persist with continuous therapy, most women manage to overcome withdrawal bleeding and totally eliminate all periods within a year.
- Cost – in some health systems, patients find they need to pay for the two hormone tablets separately.

It is easy to keep track of HRT tablets as the daily dosage is prescribed in blister packs.

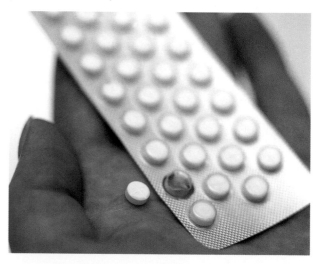

### DID YOU KNOW?
If you have had a hysterectomy, you will not need progestogen because you no longer run the risk of endometrial cancer, therefore tablets containing only oestrogen will be prescribed.

## TIBOLONE (LIVIAL)

The synthetic steroid tibolone has the properties of oestrogen, progestogen and androgen. One tablet is taken per day and it is effective in reducing the severity and frequency of hot flushes and in relieving sweating and headaches in post-menopausal women who have an intact uterus. It is not recommended for use until one year after the cessation of menstruation since vaginal bleeding may occur in women who still produce their own oestrogen.

### Advantages of tibolone
- It is given as continuous therapy.
- It is helpful for women who cannot tolerate progestogens and the withdrawal bleeds associated with them.
- It has androgenic properties that are useful for maintaining libido and energy.

### Disadvantage of tibolone
- It offers no advantage for women who have undergone a hysterectomy, either with or without oophorectomy (removal of ovaries).

## TRANSDERMAL PATCHES

Transdermal oestrogen patches contain tiny doses of oestrogen which are released through the skin. You apply the patch to a small area below your waistline or your buttocks, where the movement of your body will not cause the skin to wrinkle. The patch will need to be replaced every three to four days using a different site on your body. Progestogen is taken in pill form from days 14 to 25.

### UNLUCKY FOR SOME
It is not unnusual for women to get menopausal symptoms for many years after their periods stop. One study of Swedish women found that about 15 per cent of them were still getting hot flushes 16 years after their last period.

There is a combined oestrogen and progestogen patch available for women who still have a uterus. Again, the patch needs to be replaced twice weekly using a different site for the replacement.

### Advantages of patches
- There is a gradual, constant absorption of hormone(s) into the bloodstream.
- The patch bypasses the liver, so this is a good alternative for women with a history of liver disease.
- No need to remember to take a pill every day.

### Disadvantages of patches
- Some women find they have an allergic reaction to the adhesive, causing an itchy rash.

Transdermal patches are transparent and may wrinkle slightly when placed on the buttocks or waist.

- You may initially become fidgety and hyperactive.
- The patch adheres well enough in the shower or when swimming but may not stay on for prolonged soaks in baths.
- Sweat can also unstick a patch: women who live in hot, humid climates and athletes who perspire heavily often report the patches becomes loosened more readily.
- Occasionally, a woman's partner may complain about the aesthetics of the patch, which is generally placed on the hip, thigh or tummy. If this is a continuing problem, you might want to change to another form of HRT – or you can always change your partner!
- You will need to take progestogen tablets unless it is a combined patch.
- Cost – patches are generally more expensive than tablets and you may need to pay separately for both the patches and the progestogen tablets.

> *I was started on HRT in the form of tablets. These produced high blood pressure and headaches so I was changed to patches. They changed my life – the night sweats and flushes disappeared, as did the pain in my vagina.*
> ANNETTE (Brunei)

## HIDDEN PITFALLS

An unforeseen hazard has come to light concerning the hormone skin patches. A male doctor recently started to feel nauseous and generally unwell. When a colleague examined him the cause soon came to light: his wife's transdermal hormone patch had come adrift and was now stuck to his bottom.

*SHE* magazine Health News, March 1992

## HORMONE IMPLANTS

Implants are little pellets that are inserted under the skin in a simple surgical procedure, either at a local surgery or in a hospital outpatient department. The doctor injects a little local anaesthetic into the skin of the abdomen, a tiny cut is then made and an oestrogen pellet (about the size of an apple pip) is inserted through a tube. The tube is removed and the pellet pushed down into the fat under the skin. The opening is closed either with a stitch or a plaster.

The hormones are absorbed slowly from the pellet and a single implant can last up to nine months, according to the dose. For women who still have a uterus the implant is combined with progestogen tablets.

### Advantages of implants
- The oestrogen bypasses your liver and goes straight into the bloodstream.

The insertion of an implant in the abdomen is a quick and painless procedure.

- Convenience – once inserted, it can be forgotten. It will become apparent that it is running out with the re-emergence of menopausal symptoms.

### Disadvantages of implants

- Once inserted, the implant cannot easily be retrieved; you will have to wait until it has run its course if the dosage is incorrect.
- Unless you have had a hysterectomy, you will still be taking progestogen tablets to induce a bleed.
- The symptoms associated with the menopause appear to re-occur at shorter and shorter intervals, so that the implant has to be replaced more frequently.

## NASAL SPRAYS

A relatively new development is a once-daily nasal spray that administers oestrogen via a metered-dose pump. The hormone is absorbed through the lining of the nose and is said to mimic the way the natural hormone works. Women who have not had a hysterectomy will still need to take progestogen for at least 12 days when using this type of HRT. Nasal sprays may not be appropriate for people who have persistent nasal problems, but can still be used if you just have a cold. Blow your nose just before using the spray and try to avoid blowing it again for 15 minutes afterwards to give it time for the oestrogen to be absorbed. There is no need to take more sprays if you sneeze just after taking it.

### Advantages of nasal sprays

- The oestrogen is rapidly absorbed into the bloodstream and bypasses the liver and intestines.
- It will relieve moderate to severe symptoms in both menopausal and post-menopausal women.
- Any change in dosage can be provided by adjusting the number of sprays.
- Cost – comparable to patches or gel.

### Disadvantages of nasal sprays

- Long-term adverse effects or benefits have yet to be explored.
- Specifically, the effect on bone mineral density is still being evaluated.

## VAGINAL CREAMS

After or during the menopause many women find that vaginal dryness makes sexual intercourse less enjoyable, or even painful. This happens because of insufficient oestrogen. As we discussed earlier, the oestrogen hormones are responsible for maintaining the shape, size, flexibility and lubrication of the vagina. They hasten the flow of blood to the pelvic area during sexual arousal, and blood surges through the tissues, causing the release of fluid into the vaginal passage. This increased blood flow also makes the skin, nipples and other sensual areas respond more pleasurably to stimulation, increasing sexual response and the quality of a woman's orgasm.

If the hormone is in short supply, then the vaginal tissues become dry and less pliable: the entrance to your vagina may become so narrow that intercourse is impossible. This effect may become more obvious if your adrenal glands have been depleted by stress, and you may be aware of gradual changes as oestrogen levels diminish during the menopausal years.

### TRIAL RESULTS

A six-nation trial of oestrodiol nasal spray in 1999 showed symptoms were significantly reduced within four weeks, and that 85 per cent of women who took part in the trials elected to continue with this novel form of treatment. Tests showed that its effectiveness was equal to that of tablets.

If sexual intimacy is part of your life, either with a partner and/or through masturbation, then oestrogen in cream form can be inserted directly into the vagina using an applicator-dose to treat vaginal dryness. Even if you are taking HRT in the oral or patch form, it may be necessary to supplement with an oestrogen cream to re-lubricate your vagina.

### Advantages of vaginal creams
• Quickest way to treat vaginal dryness.
• Easily reversible.

### Disadvantages of vaginal creams
• They can be messy and it is hard to control the dosage (taking too much oestrogen can lead to overgrowth of the endometrium and the risk of developing endometrial cancer).
• The dose is too low to help with hot flushes.
• Creams should not be used directly before sexual intercourse with a man, unless he uses a condom, as he could absorb enough oestrogen through his penis over time to cause him side-effects such as breast enlargement.

## VAGINAL RINGS (ESTRING)
HRT in the form of a vaginal ring is made of silicon and is inserted high into the vagina, where it stays for three months. During this time it releases a low dose of oestrogen locally. Replacements can be inserted at three-month intervals for a period of up to two years. The ring provides a very low dosage of oestrogen only to the vagina, so many doctors believe it is safe to use vaginal rings to treat vaginal dryness or atrophy in women who have had breast cancer. Neither the woman nor her partner can feel the ring during intercourse, but if you and/or your partner find the ring uncomfortable or unacceptable, it can be removed and replaced afterwards.

### Advantages of a vaginal ring
• It can be removed easily if a problem develops.
• Oestrogen levels remain constant as long as the ring is in place.

### Disadvantages of a vaginal ring
• Some women dislike the idea of 'something up there'.
• Women who have had a hysterectomy may have trouble keeping the ring in place, especially if the vagina has been foreshortened too much in the operation.

An applicator may not have the flexibility of a tampon, but it is just as simple to insert in a vagina.

Vaginal rings are flexible and easy to handle. They are inserted high into the vagina and release a very low dose of oestrogen.

# HRT and breast cancer

## CLINICAL TRIALS

Clinical trials/studies are generally of four types:

- A *prospective study* can be placebo-controlled (where half the participants receive dummy pills), double-blinded (where neither experimenters nor the participants know the particulars of the test items), single-blinded (where the experimenters but not the participants know the particulars of the test items), or unblinded (where both experimenters and participants know the particulars of the test items).
- A *retrospective study* looks back after the effect has happened, e.g. when people develop a condition researchers will look back to discover whether any particular factor contributed to it.
- A *case-control study* is helpful in finding out the correlation between A and B factors in a rare medical condition.
- An *observational study* can be helpful in finding out a correlation between two apparently unrelated factors. A good example of this is where it was found that asbestos exposure was related to lung cancer when it was observed that many people working in an asbestos factory developed lung cancer.

In addition, researchers sometimes use *meta-analysis.* This is where similar prospective studies are pulled together and all of them are analysed as a single study. This often reveals a better picture of the medical situation.

Considerable contention and uncertainty about HRT relates to the risk of breast cancer – a disease that affected over a million people worldwide in the year 2000, one-third of whom live in Europe. The uncertainty is not helped by conflicting studies, some of which show the risk of breat cancer is reduced by HRT while others suggest a slight increase.

This controversy is clearly illustrated by the publication in the UK doctors journal the *Lancet* (1997) of a report which re-analysed the raw data of over 90 per cent of the worldwide studies of HRT and breast cancer. Individual data on nearly 53,000 women with breast cancer and just over 100,000 women without breast cancer from 51 studies in 21 countries were collected, checked and analysed. The report concluded that

> *'the risk of having breast cancer is increased in women using HRT and increases with increased duration of use. This effect is reduced after cessation of use of HRT and has largely, if not wholly, disappeared after about 5 years.'*

Reading this, you might justifiably assume that the issue is now cut and dried. Not so. Many of the studies in this report were of women who had taken oestrogen-only HRT, whereas most women these days use combined oestrogen and progestogen HRT. The breast cancers in women taking HRT were found to be smaller, more compact and less advanced than those found in women who were not taking HRT – however, that may be scant consolation for women and their families suffering the trauma of diagnosis, treatment and potential recurrence of the cancer.

Three years later, researchers at the National Cancer Institute in Rockville, Maryland, USA, released the results of a study of just under 45,000 post-menopausal women who took part in a breast cancer detection project between 1980 and 1995. The findings confirmed the potential hazards and uncertainties in the use of HRT since they showed that:

- The relative risk of developing breast cancer was 20 per cent higher for women who had taken HRT containing oestrogen than for women who had never taken HRT.
- The risk was 40 per cent higher for women who had taken oestrogen with progestogen.
- Thin women were more at risk if they took oestrogen alone.

More recent confirmation of this risk was made in 2002 when a US trial to evaluate oestrogen and progestogen use in 16,000 post-menopausal women was stopped early by the Women's Health Initiative because health risks exceeded health benefits by a small margin.

Although the number was small, women receiving this particular HRT – Prempro (a continuous combined HRT tablet marketed only in the USA) – had a higher rate of breast cancer and more adverse cardiovascular events (i.e coronary heart disease and stroke) than those receiving placebo, although there were benefits for hip fractures and bowel cancer. As the average age of the women was 63 years, it is hardly surprising there were no significant cardiovascular improvements – the degenerative effects of ageing were already apparent and ground that had been lost could not be reclaimed.

It is no surprise to find that doctors are divided about the possible links between breast cancer and HRT when faced with such complicated findings: some of them regard the risk of breast cancer as a very small one indeed; others believe the risks are unacceptable.

A baffled response to a leading article on the subject in the British Medical Journal (December 2001) summed up one doctor's desperate plea:

## SELF-EXAMINATION
It is important to know how to check your breasts yourself.

Check each breast for lumps, differences in skin texture and changes around the nipple. Feel right into each armpit.

Repeat this check in several positions and with your arms in different postures.

Try standing in front of a mirror to help you become more familiar with your breasts.

*'How is the typical working GP (or hospital clinician) to interpret supposedly 'authoritative' advice when it is so emphatically contradicted by others apparently equally well-qualified?'*

## THE WAY FORWARD FOR YOU

Before you can make an informed decision about whether to take HRT or not, you need to understand the risks as they apply to *you* and no other woman. It is certainly true that:

- Breast cancer happens whether women are taking HRT or not taking HRT.
- Breast tissue is influenced by changing levels of hormones.
- Other factors that determine the development of cancers include heredity and alcohol consumption.
- Some types of breast cancer are fast-growing and quickly fatal.
- Others develop very slowly, over 18–20 years or even longer.

It is important to consider all the risk factors that apply to you. Two possible areas related to breast cancer currently under investigation are (1) oestrogen-containing preparations, such as the contraceptive pill and HRT, and (2) dietary factors.

## Breast cancer and oestrogen

Both the contraceptive pill and HRT contain oestrogen, and it is known that oestrogen can stimulate cancer cells to grow. In theory, increasing the supply of oestrogen could trigger a breast cancer to develop – in practice, the risk of this happening appears to be a small one. Recent research looking at the contraceptive pill worldwide has revealed that:

- the incidence of breast cancer is increased slightly whilst it is taken and for up to 10 years after stopping
- more than 10 years after stopping the risk is the same as that of a woman who has never taken it
- a large number of women diagnosed with breast cancer have used the contraceptive pill during the progression of their malignant disease process.

## Breast cancer and diet

So far, the search for dietary factors implicated in breast cancer during adulthood has been disappointing. This does not preclude a possible association between breast cancer and diet *earlier* in life. The only fairly well-established dietary risk for breast cancer is alcohol – a small but consistent increase in risk has been associated with alcohol consumption.

Regular mammograms offer reassurance to women as potentially cancerous changes can be detected early.

## CHECK IT OUT

More than a million women who attended breast screening centres in the UK have volunteered to take part in 'The Million Women Study', one of the most ambitious studies of women's health ever undertaken. It aims to answer questions about links between HRT and breast cancer and heart disease. The impact of HRT and other lifestyle factors on heart disease, bone disease and joint replacement are also being investigated, as are diet, reproductive history, vitamin and mineral use and family history of illness.

> *When I was 51 years old, I took a lot of care considering the issue of HRT with my doctor, and decided to use it for severe menopausal night sweats. I took tablets for 18 months, then changed to patches for six months. Breast cancer was diagnosed just when I'd begun to feel much better.*
>
> *I underwent a lumpectomy, removal of lymph nodes, chemotherapy and radiotherapy, then a mastectomy. While I was recovering, I read two books written by Jane Plant – The Plant Programme and Your Life in their Hands and I also obtained information from the Bristol Cancer Help Centre. I decided to follow a non-dairy eating plan using lots of fresh fruit and vegetables, as well as herbs, especially sage. I eat only organic poultry and fish and take multivitamin and mineral supplements as well as vitamin C, calcium and magnesium, vitamin E and selenium. I also work out three times a week at the gym and feel on top of the world!*
>
> *Nobody in my family has ever had breast cancer and I do not think HRT alone caused it. I think that a variety of factors must exist before the cells start to go haywire and form a tumour. For me, it could have been the combination of stress and anger about my husband's redundancy, as well as working long hours in my own business, plus the HRT and high dairy intake.*
>
> JILL (Rugby)

## KNOWN RISKS

You have an increased risk of developing breast cancer if you:

- have a strong family history of breast cancer
- carry a breast cancer gene
- started your periods early (aged 10 or under) and have a late (aged 59 plus) menopause
- have no children or have them late in life (aged over 40)
- have a history of benign breast disease.

Unfortunately, you cannot do anything about most of the above, apart from being aware of them. But you can make sure you take advantage of all the health care offered to you by going for screening tests.

### Strong family history

If your mother, sister or daughter was diagnosed with breast cancer under the age of 40 years, or if you have two or more relatives diagnosed (both from one side of your family), at least one of whom is under 50 years old, or if several relatives on the same side of your family have developed breast, ovarian or colon cancer, then you have what is known as a strong family history.

This may indicate that there is a breast cancer gene in your family. Several genes have been identified that can increase breast cancer risk, but at present there are tests for only two of them: BRCA1 and BRCA2. Your risk of getting breast cancer if you carry either of these genes is about 85 per cent by the time you are 55 years old. In other words, 85 women out of 100 who carry a breast cancer gene will have developed breast cancer by the time they are 55.

### Benign breast disease

If you have a history of benign breast lumps, then you are at a very slightly increased risk of breast cancer. But 'benign breast disease' includes a wide range of different conditions, most of which do not lead to cancer. One in ten breast lumps show 'atypical hyperplasia'. This means that the cells are not cancer, but they are growing abnormally, and will increase your risk of breast cancer by four times the average.

## ADDING FUEL TO THE FIRE?

You might think that survivors of breast cancer who had taken HRT would never do so again. Indeed, there has been a longstanding recommendation that it should not be taken because of the possibility of activating the growth of another malignant tumour. Yet several quality-of-life aspects may be disrupted or worsen during treatment for cancer – menopausal symptoms such as mood swings, vaginal dryness and decreased libido are understandably common, and hot flushes and night sweats often return after treatment is completed. If this happens to you, you may find that your specialist is happy for you to take the lowest dosage of HRT, providing you are monitored regularly (e.g. every six months).

## SUMMARY

Help yourself to a decision about this adverse effect of HRT by:

- assessing *your* risk of breast cancer
- regular attendance at screening clinics
- improving your lifestyle, e.g reducing your alcohol consumption and eating more fresh fruit, bran cereals, wholemeal bread and raw salads daily.

If you are a survivor of breast cancer and are not sure whether to resume taking HRT, then:

- consider your risks and benefits
- recognize that freedom from recurrent cancer can never be guaranteed
- remember that the risk of dying from breast cancer in HRT users is 20 per cent less than that in non-users who contract the disease.

> *I had been taking HRT for 12 years when I was diagnosed with breast cancer. My family history indicated risk as my mother had died of it when she was 55, as had her two sisters. When the breast cancer specialist realized this, he arranged for me to be monitored every six months – he did not entirely approve of my taking HRT but I begged him to let me stay on it.*
>
> *In June 1997 I was clear, but in December a cancerous lump was found. I came off HRT and 10 days later had a mastectomy, followed by radiotherapy for four weeks. It was then that the absence of the HRT made itself well and truly felt – a few daytime hot flushes, but the day and night sweats were horrendous. In fact, the sweating started up at an annual check-up with the oncologist and within a few minutes I was wringing wet. I felt so miserable and asked if I could possibly go back on HRT. To my astonishment, the doctors agreed.*
>
> *I have now been back on it for over two years and feel exceptionally well. My original breast cancer specialist is now retired and his replacement seems very relaxed about it – after all, it's quality of life that counts, not quantity.*
>
> ANNE (Cornwall)

### IT'S ALL IN THE GENES

The *BRCA2* gene was first located by studying Icelandic families with a high incidence of breast cancer. Because Iceland has seen little immigration since it was first settled by a small group of Norwegians around AD900, it has a very consistent gene pool. Two Icelandic families with a history of frequent breast cancer can be traced back to a common ancestor born in 1711.

# How long can I use HRT for menopausal symptoms?

How long you continue to use HRT will depend on your symptom relief. Some women decide to take it for six months, then discontinue it for a few months and see what difference this makes to their well-being. The symptoms may return during this time, as HRT frequently just 'damps' them down, especially if they are severe, so you might decide to

- restart the therapy
- change your method of HRT, e.g from tablets to patches
- explore other solutions for your particular circumstances.

# How do I get off HRT for good?

If you stop taking the medication abruptly, you may experience symptoms of rapidly falling levels of oestrogen, such as hot flushes, migraines and vaginal dryness. These symptoms are a form of withdrawal, and it is not advisable to go 'cold turkey'. The recommended guidelines for coming off HRT are to do it gradually over three months, but before you start you should seek the advice of your doctor. For the first month substitute natural progesterone cream as described on pages 65–66 for the progestogen and reduce the oestrogen by 50 per cent. In the second month, reduce the oestrogen by 50 per cent again, and again for the third month. By the end of this month, the HRT can be safely and completely discontinued. You need to continue using the natural progesterone for the next three months.

You may find the use of natural progesterone leads to an experience of high oestrogen effects – fluid retention, tenderness and swelling of the breasts or even the appearance of scant vaginal bleeding. These effects are only temporary and will normally soon clear.

# What about taking HRT post-menopausally?

Some doctors are cautious, and believe that all HRT should be discontinued by ten years after periods have ceased, mainly because of the greater risk of breast cancer in women from their 60s onwards. Certainly, its continuing use after the age of 50 should be critically reviewed every five years. Having said that, it is not unknown for much older women to be taking it.

# Other known benefits of taking HRT

We have already looked at the benefits to be had by taking HRT for the alleviation of menopausal symptoms, and Liz has confirmed the 'feel-good' factors of fitness and energy levels post-menopausally. There are other possible long-term benefits as well. Many doctors regard HRT as an acceptable lifelong adjunct to continuing good health, especially for women at risk of any of the following: alzheimer's disease (see pages 41–42), bowel cancer (see pages 42–43), osteoporosis (see pages 44–52) and cardiovascular disease (CVD) (see pages 53–59).

*I am 84 years old and have been taking HRT for 30 years with no side-effects whatsoever. I have felt so fit and well, especially sexually – I have had three very happy relationships since my husband died 12 years ago, the last with a gentleman of 92.*

*My doctor recently refused to prescribe it again because of the recent findings about the increase in blood clotting when sitting for such long hours in an aeroplane when I visit family in Australia. I was very unhappy about this, so I changed my doctor and am now back on HRT.*

**LIZ (London)**

# Alzheimer's disease

Alzheimer's disease (also called pre-senile dementia) was named after a German doctor, Alois Alzheimer (1864–1915). He published many papers on conditions and diseases of the brain, one of which involved memory loss, behaviour and personality changes as well as a decline in cognitive abilities.

These clinical definitions in no way convey the pain and heartbreak experienced if you are intimately involved with someone who develops the disease. The actual degenerative process begins in midlife and is almost impossible to reverse.

## RISK FACTORS

You are at increased risk of developing Alzheimer's disease if you have high blood pressure and/or high levels of cholesterol (as outlined on page 53) or if one of your parents or grandparents suffered from it.

One theory is that you may be at extra risk if you undergo a dramatic loss of oestrogen at menopause, as evidenced by symptoms including memory lapses and erratic concentration. Given that the hypothalamus at the base of the brain acts as a control centre for your hormones, it would seem logical to assume that a major hormonal disturbance would be bound to have an effect on the brain.

## REDUCING THE RISK

Women who take HRT report that their ability to remember things improves almost immediately. This may be attributed to oestrogen's effect on the growth of nerve cells, improved blood flow to the brain, or due to its effect on neurotransmitters such as serotonin.

Regardless of the HRT regimen, there may be a 'critical window' in the early stages of Alzheimer's disease when HRT may prevent a progressive loss of mental faculties.

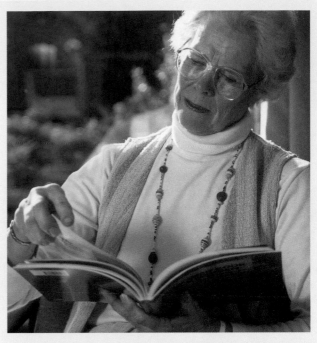

Some women continue to take HRT post-menopausally.

**Dementia** This is a deterioration of mental faculties combined with emotional disturbances resulting from an organic brain disorder, whereas Alzheimer's disease is a degenerative disease of the brain occurring in middle age and causing a progressive loss of mental faculties.

**Serotonin** An organic compound found in both animal and human tissue, especially the brain, blood serum and the lining of the digestive tract. It is capable of raising body temperature and contracting smooth muscle and has a role in changing behaviour and mood.

**Neurotransmitters** These are chemicals involved in the transmission of a nerve impulse between nerve cells.

Some experts believe that the prevention of Alzheimer's disease may become the primary reason for the prescription of HRT.

## SUMMARY

- Neither dementia nor Alzheimer's disease are necessarily part of the ageing process. It is therefore very important to consider the implications for you if your family medical history includes either of them, especially if you have high blood pressure and/or high levels of cholestrol.
- Current research indicates HRT is beneficial if you are at risk of both dementia and Alzheimer's disease.

## HRT AND DEMENTIA

Researchers in the USA studied 1,124 elderly women with an average age of 74 years, who were assessed as non-demented. During follow-up, which ranged from between 1 and 5 years they discovered that:

- of the 968 women who had never used HRT, 158 (16 per cent) developed dementia
- of the 156 women who had taken HRT at the menopause, 9 (5 per cent) developed the disorder
- none of the 23 women who were taking HRT when the study started developed dementia.

# Bowel cancer

Nearly a million people were diagnosed with bowel cancer worldwide in the year 2000, of whom just under one-third live in Europe. It is much more common in the Western world, for example, than in Asia and Africa. It is believed to be due to differences in diet. Jewish people who are Ashkenazi or of Eastern European descent, are at increased risk of bowel cancer, and it is believed that a specific gene mutation can be found in 6 per cent of this population.

Bowel cancer is the third commonest cancer in the UK (after lung and breast cancer) and the second leading cause of all-cancer death in the USA. It can occur at any age but is most common in the elderly and is rare in women under 40. The lifetime risk of developing it is around 1 in 20 for women. Nine out of ten cancers of the colon and rectum develop because of sporadic mutations in the cells lining the bowel. Sporadic mutations, which happen at random, accumulate over time and are caused by diet and the effects of advancing age.

## RISK FACTORS

One of the risk factors is a family history of the disease. Certain criteria indicating a pattern of bowel cancer throughout generations can be evaluated using the Amsterdam Criteria. These state that a person's risk of developing bowel cancer is high if their family includes:

## THE PARADOX

The risk of bowel cancer in women before the menopause is doubled if they are clinically obese, though paradoxically, after the menopause the fat tissue is an important source of oestrogen which may reduce the risk of colo-rectal cancer.

- at least three members with colon or rectal cancer
- at least two successive generations with colon or rectal cancer
- two family members with the disease who are first-degree relatives (i.e parents, brothers, sisters or children) of another family member with colon and rectal cancer
- at least one member affected at or before the age of 50.

Over the last 20 years, death rates from this disease have dropped more in women than men, and accumulating evidence suggests that post-menopausal hormone use may decrease the risk of it.

In 1976, just under 60,000 post-menopausal registered nurses in 11 US States took part in the Nurses Health Study, part of which examined the relationship between post-menopausal hormone therapy and bowel cancer. The follow-up lasted 14 years and its findings showed a reduction in risk of 35 per cent among women currently using post-menopausal hormones, but the apparent reduction substantially diminished upon cessation of therapy. This study is included in 23 observational studies which suggest a 20 per cent reduction in occurrence of bowel cancer in post-menopausal women due to HRT.

## SUMMARY

- You need to consider the implications for you if your family medical history indicates you are at risk of this cancer.
- Improving and modifying your eating lifestyle will be of benefit.
- Considerable research indicates a marked reduction in occurrence of bowel cancer due to HRT.

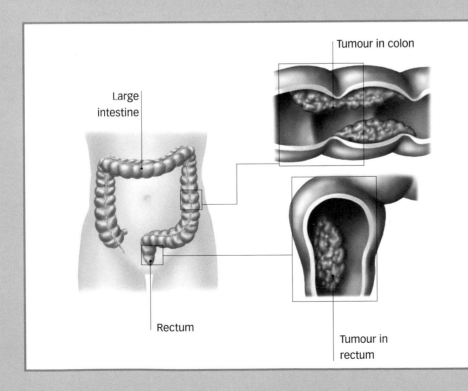

Tumour in colon

Large intestine

Rectum

Tumour in rectum

**WHERE DOES BOWEL CANCER DEVELOP?**
Bowel cancer usually affects the last part of the large intestine and the rectum.

# Osteoporosis

The skeleton is a living thing which is continually renewing itself with new bone. Bone constantly undergoes breakdown and renewal in a controlled process necessary for bone growth and repair. This is known as re-modelling.

The basic structure of your bones will not change with age, but their density and strength will reduce. This is part of the natural ageing process for men as well as women, but for some of us, the bone will be lost much faster than new bone can be formed to replace it. If this happens, bones can become so fragile that they are liable to break very easily: fractures commonly occur at the wrist, hip and spine, and the consequences can be devastating with about 20 per cent of hip fractures causing death.

This fractured bone has jagged edges. Consequently, it will take time for it to kit together.

## DID YOU KNOW?

One in every four adult white or Asian women has broken a wrist or hip bone or suffered a crush fracture of the spine by the age of 65 and half of all women have had a fracture by the time they reach the age of 75.

The condition known as osteoporosis is a worldwide disease, as evidenced by the formation of support, information and research organizations for osteoporosis in 70 countries. Racial origin influences a woman's risk of brittle bones – women of African, Aboriginal or Mediterranean extraction are unlikely to suffer osteopororis because they usually possess thicker bones and have reached a greater bone mass at skeletal maturity. On the other hand Caucasian, Asian or Oriental women possess generally thinner bones and lower bone mass, and therefore face a greater risk.

Osteoporosis can begin anywhere from 5 to 20 years before the menopause when oestrogen levels are still high. It accelerates for a few years at the menopause or if the ovaries are surgically removed or become non-functioning, as can happen after a hysterectomy. At such times, the rate of bone loss will increase from 2 to 5 per cent a year. However, for some women its foundations may well have been laid many years earlier by a diet grossly deficient in calcium, or a demanding athletic schedule which inhibited ovulation.

Osteoporosis is a silent disease which goes unnoticed and is usually painless in the early stages. Because you cannot see your bones, you may not know there is anything amiss until you break your hip, spine or wrist due to a minor bump or fall. Other symptoms include:

- loss in height
- a curving spine
- acute and unexplained back pain.

Osteoporosis can lead to a dramatic loss of height, severe curvature of the spine, chronic pain and permanent disability. It can literally devastate lives, and everyday activities which we all take for granted can become impossible.

## RISK FACTORS

The following place you at high risk of osteoporosis:

- Very early menopause before the age of 45 – this causes early loss of oestrogen because your ovaries stop working.
- An early menopause before the normal age of 50 – early loss of oestrogen is likely, and certain if your ovaries are removed.
- Long-term use of high-dose corticosteroids (for conditions such as arthritis and asthma). Do not stop taking them – your doctor may be able to adjust your dosage to compensate for bone loss.
- Irregular or infrequent menstruation – this can happen naturally or be caused by over-exercising, if you are a dancer, or suffer from anorexia nervosa or bulimia. This results in low oestrogen levels similar to menopause, regardless of age.
- Disorders of the digestion that cause malabsorption problems, such as coeliac disease, Crohn's disease or gastric surgery.
- Heavy smoking – this can damage bone-building cells and cause an early menopause.
- Low calcium intake – consumption of milk and dairy products maintain bone density.
- Heavy drinking – alcohol abuse destroys bone.
- Immobility – bones need exercise to remain strong, so those who are bed- and wheelchair-bound are more at risk.
- Lack of sunshine – exposure to sunlight is necessary for vitamin D production which is essential for bone health as a bone hardener.

Much of the variation in bone mineral mass and the incidence of osteoporosis can be ascribed to genetic differences between individuals, and therefore a family history of osteoporosis puts you more at risk of having fractures later in life. If you are aware of a history of osteoporosis in your family you would be well advised to ask for bone density testing.

*I began suffering very strong back pain in 1995, and thought it was just the 'ageing' effect. But as time went on, my agility and mobility plummeted, and I had to depend more and more on my family for help. Visits to the doctor led to pain-killers, then stronger pain-killers, and I lost three precious years before I was found to have suffered severe loss of bone density.*

CARMEN (Spain)

## DRINK MORE MILK

In 1994, a cross-sectional study of 284 women aged 44–74 living in Cambridge, UK, revealed that frequent milk consumption before the age of 25 was associated with 5 per cent higher hip bone mineral density in middle-aged women and older women.

## DID YOU KNOW?

A child's skeleton is replaced every two years, an adult's every 7–10 years. After bones have stopped growing in length at the age of 16–18 years, they still increase in density. After about the age of 35 they begin to deteriorate.

## DIAGNOSIS

The best way to identify osteoporosis in its early form is a test using X-rays called dual energy X-ray absorptiometry (DXA), often referred to as a DXA scan. This can detect tiny amounts of bone loss of 1–3 per cent and regular yearly scans allow the rate of loss to be calculated.

At present, this method of bone density scanning is the most accurate and reliable method of assessing the strength of your bones. A DXA machine would usually scan your lower spine and one hip. Other areas which can also be assessed include your forearm and heel.

### BONE DENSITY TESTING
Whatever is used to predict osteoporotic fractures, a measure of bone mass is only valuable if associated with a clinical comment and opinion from a registered medical doctor experienced in bone mass measurement.

Bone density is then compared to young, healthy adult measurements.

DXA machines are large, static pieces of equipment. A less expensive diagnostic method uses a portable ultrasound machine which can assess your bone structure and strength, usually of your heel bone (calcaneus), wrist or finger. Heel ultrasound is also useful in predicting your osteoporotic fracture risk around the time of your menopause and of Colles (wrist) fracture in your early post-menopausal years.

## REDUCE YOUR RISK BY INVESTING IN YOUR BONES

### Your bones need calcium
Calcium accounts for approximately 67 per cent of bone weight and bones act as a storage bank for calcium. If the amount of calcium in your blood falls below a certain level, your body will take its calcium needs from your bones. This calcium withdrawn from your bones is used for other important functions of your body, i.e. those of the heart, muscles, blood and nerves.

Clearly, it is important to maintain your intake of dietary calcium and the chart opposite sets out ways in which you can increase this. However, it is also important to be aware of the way that other substances in foods and drinks can affect your calcium levels.

Substances that can reduce calcium absorption (when taken in large quantities) include:

- Phytates – present in fibre, particularly unprocessed bran
- Tannins – present in tea
- Oxalate – present in spinach
- Caffeine – present in coffee, tea and cola drinks
- Phosphates without calcium, for example fizzy, canned drinks

# Increasing your calcium intake

## Daily requirement

*before menopause* 1,000mg

*after menopause* 1,500mg

*Calcium content of common foods in milligrams per 100g (approx 3½oz) of food*

### DAIRY

| | |
|---|---|
| Cheese | |
| *Cheddar* | 800 |
| *Cottage* | 80 |
| *Danish blue* | 580 |
| *Edam* | 740 |
| *Parmesan* | 1,220 |
| *Processed* | 700 |
| *Spread* | 510 |
| Cream | 79 |
| Egg (whole) | 52 |
| Egg (yolk) | 130 |
| Milk (semi-skimmed) | |
| 0.5 litres (1pint) | 702 |
| Milk (skimmed) | |
| 0.5 litres (1pint) | 705 |
| Yogurt – low fat | 180 |
| Ice cream | 134 |

### VEGETABLES

| | |
|---|---|
| Beans, haricot | 180 |
| Beans, kidney | 140 |
| Broccoli | 100 |
| Cabbage | 53 |
| Chick peas | 140 |
| Greens – kale | 98 |
| Olives in brine | 61 |
| Parsley | 330 |
| Peas | 31 |
| Spinach | 600 |
| Spring onions | 140 |
| Watercress | 220 |
| Baked potato (large) | 24 |
| Baked beans | |
| (350g/12¼oz can) | 239 |

### MEAT AND FISH

Meat and fish contain very small amounts of calcium. Most pies and fish in batter contain calcium in the flour. Canned pilchards and sardines, sprats and whitebait contain calcium in the bones.

| | |
|---|---|
| *Prawns* | 150 |
| *Crab (canned)* | 120 |
| *Pilchards (canned)* | 300 |
| *Salmon (canned)* | 93 |
| *Sardines (canned)* | 460–550 |
| *Sprats (fried)* | 620–710 |
| *Whitebait (fried)* | 860 |
| *Fish paste* | 280 |
| *Steamed scallops* | 120 |

### FRUIT

| | |
|---|---|
| Apricots, dried | 92 |
| Blackcurrants | 60 |
| Currants | 95 |
| Figs | 280 |
| Lemon, whole | 110 |
| Rhubarb | 100 |
| Orange (1 large) | 99 |

### NUTS

| | |
|---|---|
| Almonds | 250 |
| Brazils | 180 |
| Peanuts, roasted and | |
| salted | 61 |
| Sesame seeds | 870 |

### DRINKS (DRY WEIGHT)

| | |
|---|---|
| Cocoa powder | 130 |
| Coffee, ground | 130 |
| instant | 160 |
| Malted milk drink | 230 |
| Tea, Indian | 430 |

### FLOUR AND BAKED FOODS

| | |
|---|---|
| Bread, white or brown | 100 |
| Cake, sponge | 140 |
| rock (individual fruit cake) | 390 |
| Flour, plain | 210–40 |
| self-raising | 350 |
| Soya flour | 210–40 |
| Wheat bran | 110 |

### COOKING INGREDIENTS

| | |
|---|---|
| Curry powder | 640 |
| Mustard, dry | 330 |
| Pepper | 130 |
| Salt | 230 |
| Stock cubes | 180 |
| Yeast, dried | 80 |

Substances that increase the loss of calcium in your urine include:

- Salt – a high salt intake increases urinary calcium loss
- Protein – excessive intake, i.e more than four times a day, of protein from animal sources
- Caffeine – coffee, tea and other caffeine-containing drinks cause increased output of urine, therefore increased loss of calcium.

## Your bones need vitamin D

Vitamin D enhances calcium absorption. It is present in apples, watercress, tuna, salmon and herring. But the best source of vitamin D is sunlight which increases vitamin D production in the skin.

## Your bones need magnesium

Magnesium is essential for the proper metabolism of calcium, and your bones need twice as much magnesium as calcium if the biochemistry of your bone formation is to run smoothly. Good sources are dark green vegetables, apples, seeds, nuts, figs and lemons, as well as whole grains such as brown rice, whole wheat and whole rye.

## Your bones need vitamins C, B6 and K

Vitamin C is crucial for bone formation as it produces collagen (fibrous matter) which makes up some 90 per cent of the bone matrix. Good sources of vitamin C include citrus fruits (oranges, lemons, limes), green and leafy vegetables, berries, potatoes, sweet potatoes and yams.

Vitamin B6 appears to increase the strength of connective tissue in bones. It is found in wholegrains, fish, nuts, bananas and avocados.

Vitamin K is known primarily for its effect on blood clotting and it helps to harden bone – the best source is green vegetables.

**DID YOU KNOW?**
Gardening boosts self-esteem, builds confidence and will soon be prescribed by doctors.
*Thrive (formerly the Society for Horticultural Therapy)*

## Your bones need exercise

The best type of exercise to strengthen bones is weight-bearing exercise. Your bones need to be loaded as you move. Good weight-bearing exercises include walking, jumping, ice-skating, running, skipping, ball sports, running up and down stairs, digging the garden, aerobics and tennis. You need to aim to exercise for 20 minutes a day, three times a week.

## WHAT ELSE CAN BE DONE?

Osteoporosis can be treated. If you are diagnosed with osteoporosis, or have sustained fractures from the disease, you should be aware that it is never too late to begin treatment. There are a range of medications and treatments available which have been shown to be effective in slowing or halting bone loss and helping to prevent fractures. These treatments include the following options.

## Bisphosphonates

This relatively new class of drugs is a non-hormonal type of treatment. Bisphosphonates allow bone-building cells to work more effectively, consequently resulting in increased bone density.

Three bisphosphonates currently available are:

- Risedronate (trade name Actonel) – shown to increase bone density and reduce the risk/frequency of fractures at the spine and hip
- Alendronate (trade name Fosamax) – shown to increase bone density and reduce the frequency of fractures at the hip and spine
- Etidronate (trade name Didronel) – shown to increase bone density and reduce the risk of fracture in the spine but not the hip.

## Selective oestrogen receptor modulators (SERMs)

SERMs are a special class of drug with many features similar to oestrogen in HRT. However, they differ in

### FRACTURED BONES IN EUROPE

A European audit of osteoporotic fractures published in December 2001 disclosed the following rates per 10,000 people:

| | | | |
|---|---|---|---|
| Sweden | 20.1 | Italy | 13.6 |
| Denmark | 17.9 | Greece | 12.3 |
| Germany | 16.4 | France | 9.1 |
| UK | 14.4 | Portugal | 8.2 |

### DID YOU KNOW?

The bones of elite athletes and dancers are their 'tools of the trade' and very intensive training may actually be damaging to bone. Training and performance programmes require awareness of individual physiques and nutrient requirements. Ultimate success depends on a supremely healthy skeleton supporting that body.

that they do not stimulate the breast and uterine tissues and, as a result, SERMs have the positive effect of oestrogen on bone without increasing the risk of breast and uterine cancer. However, they have no effect on hot flushes, so are of little help if you are struggling with this symptom. They are more promising if you want to counteract the long-term health risk of osteoporosis without taking a hormone that carries the risk of breast cancer.

The SERM called raloxifene (trade name Evista) is a once-daily tablet. It has been shown to increase bone density and reduce the risk of bone fractures in the spine. The long-term effect of Evista on the risk of breast cancer is unknown at present.

## Hormone replacement therapy (HRT)

HRT is the only drug therapy currently available for the treatment of osteoporosis in women regardless of whether they have had a fracture or not. Your bones can benefit from HRT but only if it is taken long-term. The Framingham Study (a long-term American health research project begun in 1948) revealed in 1993 that:

- Only women who had taken HRT for at least seven years had significantly higher bone mineral density than women who had not taken it.

- The bone mineral density of HRT users declined rapidly as soon as they stopped taking HRT.
- Even seven years of therapy might be insufficient to protect women 75 years and older from fracture.

## Calcium supplements

These may be advisable if you cannot obtain your recommended daily intake through food and drink (see the chart on page 47 for the calcium content of common foods).

## Vitamin D/calcitonins

Vitamin D supplements are recommended for people with vitamin D deficiency as a result of poor diet or limited exposure to sunlight, for example if you are aged over 65 and housebound or living in an institution. Remember, however, that excessive exposure to sun can cause skin cancer.

Calcitrol (trade names Rocaltrol and Calcijex) helps to increase the amount of calcium absorption in the gut and increase the amount of calcium that enters the bone.

*My mother is only 69 years old, yet she has a hunchback (kyphosis) that results in severe back pain which prevents her from sitting for long periods of time. She has lost 6cm in height, has problems finding suitable clothing and can wear only sports shoes to prevent possible falls. She was diagnosed as suffering from severe osteoporosis nearly 20 years after the onset of her menopause. I am not taking any chances – I take HRT and daily calcium supplements, and undergo bone density testing every two years.*

SARAH (Israel)

## SIMPLE SOLUTIONS

In 2001, a randomized controlled trial in Melbourne, Australia, explored three interventions to prevent falls among older people with participants aged 70 years and over, half of whom lived alone. The three interventions were group-based exercise, home hazard management and vision improvement. Balance measures improved significantly among the exercise group, but the strongest effect was observed for all three interventions, producing an estimated 14 per cent reduction in the annual fall rate.

In this picture you can clearly see the effects of osteoporosis on the spine.

## FALLS AND THEIR PREVENTION

Most of the fractures associated with osteoporosis are caused by falls. A third of people over the age of 60 have a fall at least once a year and although not all falls are serious, many result in fractures, especially in older women with osteoporosis.

The chart below describes some of the most common reasons for falls and provides suggestions for ways to prevent such falls.

### WHO IS AT RISK?

Most hip fractures occur in people aged over 80 years with associated high morbidity and mortality. It is therefore desirable to identify those individuals at greatest risk because that risk can be roughly halved with effective treatment.
*Ignac Fogelman, Professor of Nuclear Medicine, Guy's Hospital, London*

### COMMON REASONS FOR FALLS

| Reasons | Prevention |
| --- | --- |
| Poor balance caused by weak muscles, low blood pressure, ear problems or other conditions | • *Exercise keeps muscles strong and improves balance* |
| Poor eyesight making it harder to notice hazards, such as a trailing cord or a bump in the footpath | • *Make sure you have good lighting in your home*<br>• *Get an annual eye test*<br>• *Avoid glare by wearing good-quality sunglasses* |
| Footwear | • *Ensure your shoes are well-fitting* |
| Hazards at home (most falls occur in the home) | • *Floor surfaces – mats, carpets, rugs should lie flat without curled-up edges*<br>• *Make sure electrical cords are not hanging where you walk* |
| Lighting | • *Have clear lighting in all areas in your home with easily accessible switches* |
| Bathroom | • *Have railings fitted to help you in/out of the shower/bathtub and when using the toilet*<br>• *Use non-slip mats to avoid slippery wet surfaces* |
| Hazards outside the home | • *Be aware of uneven pavements, slippery shopping centre floors, steep kerbs, etc.*<br>• *Keep your garden free of clutter including fallen branches and hosepipes* |

## BATHROOM SAFETY

There are some simple precautions you can take to avoid falls in the bathroom. Install hand rails for getting in and out of the bath and always use a non-slip bathmat.

## SUMMARY

If you have experienced an early menopause; prolonged amenorrhea (i.e. abnormal suppression or absence of menstruation other than because of pregnancy); if you have a family history of osteoporosis or are taking corticosteroids, then a bone scan will be helpful in reaching a decision about treatment.

Explore all your options for maintaining healthy bones for the rest of your life – if you care for your bones, then your bones will take care of you.

*At the age of 49 I had a full hysterectomy as a result of cancer. In my late 50s I broke several ribs falling over a box, and broke several others ten years later. Then in 1995, at the age of 63, I fell off a ladder and broke a leg, fractured my sternum, cracked my collar-bone, chipped an elbow and again broke four ribs. It was only then I was diagnosed with osteoporosis when a bone density scan showed I was at extreme risk of fracture of my hips and spine.*

*My doctor put me on a programme of daily medication to build up my bone mass which I've kept up for the last four years. Even so, my bones are still extremely brittle: last week when bringing in the groceries from the car, I used my little finger to lift a plastic supermarket bag containing two 1-litre cartons of milk and my finger snapped.*

*For me, living with osteoporosis means:*
- *I must be careful all the time*
- *I must not hurry, especially on uneven surfaces and on rainy days*
- *I must keep my dog, Gemmi, on a short leash when I walk her each day so that I don't get tangled up and trip over*
- *I must not wear high heels*
- *Because of its effects on bone density, I must limit alcohol or better still, abstain*
- *I must carry in groceries in small amounts, making several trips up 17 stairs*
- *I must no longer dig the vegetable garden or climb or stretch up to trim trees*
- *I must only spring clean things I can reach from floor level*

*Most of all, it means not being able to run around with my grandchildren – I'm the person sitting on the beach minding the shoes, instead of exploring the rockpools.*

**BONNIE (New Zealand)**

# HRT and heart disease

If you hold out your hand, palm upwards, you will see bluish veins visible under the fine skin of your wrist – these are part of an intricate vascular system circulating blood throughout your body.

A healthy blood supply flows freely, but sometimes blockages can occur (as in a blood clot) or the veins become furred up (like the inside of a kettle) and if one of these happens to you, you are at risk of suffering either a stroke or a heart attack. These two conditions are part of the group of disorders known as cardiovascular disease (CVD).

Heart and circulatory disease, or cardiovascular disease (CVD) includes all diseases of the heart and blood vessels. The two main diseases in this category are coronary heart disease (CHD) and stroke, but CVD also includes congenital heart disease (i.e. heart deformities present at birth), valvular heart disease and a range of other diseases of the heart and blood vessels. Both CHD and stroke have a similar cause – a blockage in an artery.

Coronary heart disease (CHD) comes in two main forms: angina and heart attack – the latter is also known as a myocardial infarction.

- Angina is caused by a narrowing of the blood vessels to the heart muscle. It is experienced as a pain in the chest brought on by exercise or emotion. It can be mild or severe and generally lasts less than 10 minutes.
- A heart attack causes similar pain but lasts longer and can be fatal. A heart attack results when a blood vessel is entirely blocked by a blood clot.

Cardiovascular disease is a more common cause of morbidity and mortality for women in most countries

**High blood pressure** Blood pressure means the pressure of the blood in your arteries, i.e. the tubes that take blood away from your heart to the rest of your body. High blood pressure happens if the walls of the larger arteries lose their elasticity and become rigid, and the smaller vessels contract (become narrower). People with high blood pressure run a higher risk of having a stroke or heart attack.

**Peripheral arterial disease** This happens when the arteries which supply blood to the legs become narrowed or completely blocked off. Other arteries, e.g. those supplying blood to the heart and neck, are also likely to be affected.

**Diabetes and heart disease** These are two of the world's most common chronic diseases. More than 10 million people in Europe have diabetes.

**Blood cholesterol** There are two types of cholesterol: dietary and blood. Dietary is contained in food, while blood cholesterol is the amount circulating in the body. Cholesterol is manufactured in the liver and can be deposited in the artery walls by a process called atherosclerosis, which leads to narrowing and hardening of the arteries and then to heart disease.

of the world than osteoporosis and cancer combined. It is unusual for cardiovascular events to occur before women are in their 60s.

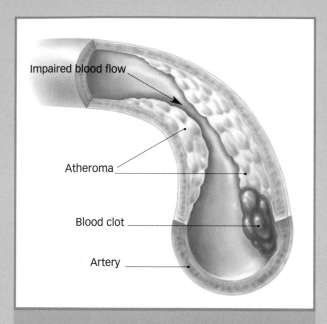

Impaired blood flow

Atheroma

Blood clot

Artery

## BLOCKED ARTERIES

The process of coronary heart disease (CHD) begins when the coronary arteries become narrowed by a gradual build-up of fatty material (atheroma) within their walls.

High blood pressure or high cholesterol levels in midlife, and in particular the combination of these risks, increases the risk of Alzheimer's disease in later life by inducing atherosclerosis and thus impairing blood flow to the brain.

## DID YOU KNOW?

Every year, more than 500,000 people die in the European Union as a result of using tobacco, with an average loss of 21 years in life expectancy.

## RISK FACTORS

The following factors place you at high risk of CVD (cardiovascular disease):

- High blood pressure – the most important risk factor for a stroke
- A family history of heart disease
- Obesity – this is defined as having a body mass index (BMI) of 30 or higher. A BMI of 26 or higher classifies you as overweight (see the formula for measuring your BMI on page 56)
- A sedentary lifestyle
- Cigarette smoking – consistently associated with peripheral arterial disease
- Psychosocial factors – stressful situations, depression and social isolation have been linked to increased risk
- Diabetes
- High blood cholesterol – associated with cardiovascular disease.

The combined effect of two or more risk factors is more powerful than any one risk factor, and some risk factors commonly occur together. For example, screening for diabetes may be appropriate in women with high blood pressure.

## THE HEART OF THE MATTER

As we get older, our pattern of risk changes. On average, women acquire heart disease about ten years later than men. Coronary heart disease rates become more similar in men and women as they age but this reflects a deceleration in male rates of heart disease during middle age, rather than an acceleration in women's post-menopausal rates.

A huge amount of research has been conducted on men and heart disease, but CVD in women is under-researched and under-diagnosed, so that comparatively little is known about it. For years it has been assumed

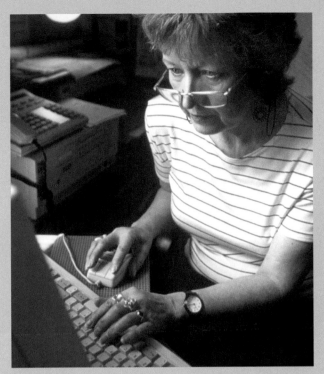

A sedentary lifestyle can place you at risk of heart disease, If your job requires you to sit at a desk all day then make sure that the rest of your life isn't so sedentary.

## CVD IS LARGELY PREVENTABLE

This has been successfuly demonstrated by a community-wide heart health programme carried out in the Finnish region of North Karelia, where over a period of 20 years CVD mortality fell by around 70 per cent.

## TOO MANY BROKEN HEARTS

CVD accounts for more than half of all deaths in Europe of people aged under 75, with a total of four million lives taken every year. The Greeks smoke the most and have the biggest problem with CVD; the Portuguese exercise the least and have the highest death rate in the EU from stroke; the Irish are the most likely to die from coronary heart disease (CHD).

women are protected from heart disease as long as oestrogen is produced, because this has a beneficial effect on blood cholesterol metabolism. It therefore followed that women lost that protection after the menopause because of the loss of oestrogen, hence the increased risk.

As discussed in Chapter 1, women do indeed lose oestrogen during the menopausal years – approximately 40 per cent of it – but it continues to be produced in variable quantities for up to 20 years after the menopause.

The observation that the progression of CVD in women is more rapid after the menopause led to the hypothesis that maintaining oestrogen levels with HRT could prevent it. Indeed, since the 1970s, more than 30 case-control and prospective studies have reported less heart disease in women using oestrogen.

*My life changed completely when I was 50 years old. I was sent abroad on business, and on my return, was hospitalized for investigations into persistent vomiting and diarrhoea. At the time I smoked and was also stressed out with my job.*

*I had a stroke in hospital which the doctor blamed on HRT – I don't think this was true as I had been on it for five years with no problems. Not long afterwards, I suffered my first bout of epilepsy.*

*In the next couple of years, I became very depressed, confused and moody and was so relieved when my doctor again prescribed HRT – I am now 61 years old, have been taking it for nine years and all of my symptoms have vanished.*

**LAURA (Bristol)**

# Body mass index

The amount of body fat you carry may be more significant than your weight alone. The Body Mass Index (BMI) expresses the relationship between a person's weight and height. It is calculated as weight in kilograms, divided by height in metres squared. The best way to determine a good weight range for you is to use the BMI formula – you will find a calculator helpful in working it out. Your BMI should fall somewhere between 18 and 25. To be either below 18 or above 25 is to put your health at risk.

Watch your weight during this menopausal transition, as any excess could affect your heart.

## CALCULATING YOUR BODY MASS INDEX

Here are 2 ways to work out your BMI:

**Method 1:**

1. Your weight (in kilograms) is X.
2. Multiply your height (in metres) by your height (in metres). This is Y.
3. Divide X by Y.

**Method 2:**

1. Multiply your present weight (in pounds) by 704. This is X.
2. Multiply your height (in inches) by your height (in inches). This is Y.
3. Divide X by Y.

*Example:*

Let's say you are 5 feet 4" (64 inches) tall and weigh 142 pounds.

Multiply 142 by 704 – this totals 99,968.

Next, multiply 64 by 64 for a total of 4,096.

Divide 99,968 by 4,096 to result in a BMI of around 24.

You are within a healthy range, although near the high end, and you should be aware that if you gain 10 pounds, your BMI will be in the unhealthy range.

However, one meta-analysis of 22 randomized trials before 1997 that compared HRT with placebo, no therapy or vitamins/minerals in predominantly healthy post-menopausal women showed no overall cardioprotective effect of HRT.

The study most often quoted to back up these claims formed part of the Nurses Health Study (see page 43) which found a decreased risk of major or fatal heart disease in oestrogen users. But closer examination of the coronary risk factors of this study reveals that this decrease had little to do with the fact that the women were taking HRT – it had far more to do with the reality of their composition as a group, for they were a self-selected group of healthy women with less severe

Severe varicose veins are a predisposing factor in the risk of developing a blood clot.

vascular risk in the first place and they were women who had a commitment to preventative medicine in general.

Oestrogen was not keeping these women healthy – healthy women were taking oestrogen. And indeed all women in HRT studies are generally better educated, comfortably off and enjoy healthier lifestyles.

## HRT SEEMS NOT TO PROTECT WOMEN FROM FURTHER HEART ATTACKS

This was the conclusion in 1998 of the first randomized controlled trial large enough to examine the effects of HRT on CVD outcomes. Researchers from 18 medical centres in the USA contributed to a study of 2,763 post-menopausal women with known heart disease whose health was followed for an average of four years. The Heart and Oestrogen/Progestogen Replacement Study (HERS) found that the overall rate of cardiovascular events did not differ between the women taking HRT and those taking placebo.

However, an increased risk of venous thromboembolic disease was observed consistently during each year of HERS.

Past perceptions about appropriate indications for the use of HRT were based almost entirely on clinical experience and observational data. These perceptions are being questioned as new knowledge emerges as a result of clinical trials.

> My hot flushes persisted for five to six years after the menopause, even though I was taking HRT. It is difficult to say what benefits it has bought me – my skin has always been clear, and my hair glossy, but as I smoke, I think it has protected my heart.
>
> JEAN (Cheltenham)

## DID YOU KNOW?
One clinical trial showed that a 'Mediterranean diet' supplemented with alpha-linoleic acid found in seeds and nuts significantly reduced the risk of recurrent coronary events in patients with heart disease.

## VITAMIN E

A study by scientists at Cambridge University and Papworth Hospital, UK, in 1996 found that a daily dose of vitamin E reduced the risk of having a heart attack by 75 per cent. This 18-month double-blind controlled trial involved 2000 patients with coronary atherosclerosis (see box, page 53). The number of heart attacks in the group taking the vitamin E was a quarter of that in the group taking placebo.

If you smoke you are more at risk of heart disease.

## CURRENT PERCEPTIONS

Although current thinking on this issue is that HRT protects against coronary disease, the randomized clinical trials reported so far have shown no benefit for reducing further coronary events. Similarly, although it is said that, unlike oral contraceptives, HRT does not increase the risk of venous thromboembolism (a blood clot), clinical trials have confirmed a three-fold increased risk of venous thromboembolism in women taking HRT.

The risk of blood clot appears to be at its greatest during the first year of use and predisposing factors are:

- a personal or family history of venous thromboembolism
- recent surgery or trauma
- obesity
- severe varicose veins
- prolonged immobilization.

Heart disease is a degenerative disease linked to lifestyle factors and when it occurs it is because problems have been building up for years.

## REDUCING YOUR RISK

There are many dietary and lifestyle changes that you can make to reduce your risk of cardiovascular disease.

- Include more oily fish, nuts, seeds and oils in your meals. The essential fatty acids in these foods are important for the prevention of heart disease. Eating fish three times a week reduces the risk of CVD as fish oils lower cholesterol, thin your blood and reduce the risk of narrowing of the arteries.
- Try to stay within an appropriate weight range for your height and frame.
- Stop smoking cigarettes and avoid 'passive' smoking situations.

## ISCHAEMIC HEART DISEASE

'Ischaemia' means an inadequate supply of blood, and is a consequence of the gradual narrowing of the coronary arteries which supply the blood and oxygen to the muscles of the heart.

You can maintain muscle mass with these handheld weights by training for at least 1 hour a week.

## RAW FOOD FOR A HEALTHY HEART

An ambitious study between 1973 and 1979 recruited 11,000 British men and women from among the customers of health food shops and other people with an interest in health foods and vegetarianism.

Its aim was to examine the relationship between six dietary factors – a vegetarian diet and consumption of wholemeal bread, bran cereals, nuts and dried fruit, fresh fruit and raw salad – and mortality for which associations with diet have been suggested.

The most significant association revealed after a 17-year follow-up to 1995 that daily consumption of raw salad was associated with a 26 per cent reduction in death from ischaemic heart disease (see box, opposite), slightly greater than that for fresh fruit (24 per cent).

- Eat more soya. Soya beans are a complete protein as they contain all eight essential amino acids.
- Eat more fresh vegetables and fruit as well as dried fruit. Fibre in potatoes, carrots, apples, beans and oats binds up the cholesterol and carries it out of your body.
- Take vitamin E supplements.
- If you have a disability which prevents you from taking active exercise, try to arrange regular physiotherapy, massage and hydrotherapy sessions.

## SUMMARY

Help yourself to a decision about this issue by

- assessing your risk of CVD
- reducing risk by eliminating two or more of your risk factors
- improving your lifestyle and adopting healthier eating habits
- protecting your heart with regular weight-bearing exercise
- recognizing that HRT cannot prevent CVD.

Remember, if you have already suffered a heart attack or stroke, HRT will not protect you against another occurrence.

# The special case of diabetes

Diabetes is one of the world's two most common chronic diseases, and more than 10 million people in Europe have the disease. Diabetic women are at greatly increased risk of developing ischaemic heart disease.

Diabetes mellitis is a condition in which the amount of glucose (sugar) in the blood is too high because the body cannot use it properly.

Glucose comes from the digestion of starchy foods such as bread, rice, potatoes, chapatis, yams and plantain, as well as sugar and other sweet foods. It is also produced in the body in the liver.

There are two main types of diabetes :

- **Type 1 diabetes, also known as insulin-dependent diabetes, usually appears before the age of 40**
- **Type 2 diabetes, also known as non-insulin diabetes, is more common among women after, rather than prior to, the menopause.**

Type 1 diabetes develops if the body is unable to produce any insulin (a hormone produced by the pancreas) and it

Bread is a universal staple food containing complex carbohydrates.These are an important source of energy.

is treated by insulin injections. Dietary changes are essential. Type 2 diabetes (late onset in midlife or older) develops when the body can still produce some insulin, but not enough, or when the insulin that is produced does not work properly. It is treated either by diet and exercise alone; by diet, exercise and tablets; or by diet, exercise and insulin injections.

The risk of death from CVD is five times greater in women aged 50–60 years who have diabetes than in women of the same age who do not. Coronary heart disease (CHD) is a major cause of morbidity and mortality in post-menopausal women with type 2 (non-insulin-dependent) diabetes. Furthermore, the Framingham Study (as mentioned on pages 49–50) showed a sixfold increase of sudden cardiac death in female compared with male diabetic patients.

One British study in 1998 revealed that type 2 diabetic post-menopausal women were 30 per cent less likely to be prescribed HRT, compared with non-diabetic women, even though its use was associated with a 50 per cent reduction in CHD. The reason for this reluctance to

## DIABETES AND OSTEOPOROSIS

Women with with type 1 diabetes have reduced bone density which can be demonstrated after a few years of insulin treatment. While it is known that insulin is important for the growth of bone cells and mineral metabolism, the exact mechanism of the osteopenia of diabetes is not fully understood.

Type 2 diabetic women have increased bone turnover but normal bone density.

prescribe is unclear but it seems to be driven by a perception that HRT will increase thromboembolic events and cause a deterioration in glucose tolerance.

In the future, it may well be that all women with diabetes should take HRT to reduce their risk of CVD. However, the appropriate studies have not yet been done. Indeed, there are no long-term studies of women with diabetes, and no studies at all on women with type 1 diabetes.

Type 1 diabetes is treated by insulin injections, but you may not need injections if you suffer from Type 2 diabetes.

## A surgical menopause

If you have had a hysterectomy (removal of the womb) and/or oophorectomy (removal of the ovaries) you are likely to be prescribed hormone replacement therapy following surgery. This will be for various reasons, depending on your age and on why you needed the surgery. HRT would be recommended for you:

- If you are a young woman (20–30 years of age) having a hysterectomy and oophorectomy, because you are likely to experience very severe menopausal symptoms.
- If you are young (20–30 years of age) and having an oophorectomy, because you will experience an artificial menopause and have increased risk of osteoporosis.
- If you are near to menopause (45–50 years of age) undergoing hysterectomy because you may experience menopausal symptoms.
- If you are near to menopause (48–52 years of age) and undergoing hysterectomy and oophorectomy.

In addition, if you are near to your menopause, post-menopausal and/or disabled, HRT would be recommended, not only because of menopausal symptoms but because of the added difficulties of possible osteoporosis.

### DIABETES AND HRT

There is no evidence that short-term treatment using HRT to relieve menopausal symptoms is unsafe for women with diabetes. In most women there is no effect on insulin requirements but occasionally a little more insulin may be needed to maintain good control of glucose levels. The use of HRT on a long-term basis is much more controversial.

### ONE IN FOUR

In 25 per cent of women who have had their wombs removed, the ovaries become less efficient and premature menopause sets in within two years. No one is quite certain why this happens but it could be due to a loss of blood supply to the ovaries or because they become encased in thick adhesions following hysterectomy.

# The missing hormone – natural progesterone

In the early 1900s, research into the mysteries of women's hormones first revealed the existence of oestrogen. Further investigations identified a second hormone which was necessary to maintain a successful pregnancy: this was named progesterone (i.e pro-gestation).

Since then, research into menopausal problems has concentrated almost exclusively on the perceived loss of oestrogen, and little attention has been paid to the decline in progesterone, because it was believed that its main purpose was to help reproductive function.

There is now a body of opinion that has challenged this assumption. It is spearheaded by a doctor who has contributed hugely to our knowledge of hormones by bringing the issue of the use of progesterone before the medical world.

## IN THE BEGINNING...

In 1994 an American doctor addressed 125 fellow medical practitioners at a meeting in a London hospital. His topic was the hormone progesterone.

A family practitioner for 30 years, John Lee had become increasingly concerned about his ageing osteoporotic patients who were unable to take oestrogen because they already had breast cancer, diabetes or vascular disorders. He realized he could encourage them to adopt a more healthy lifestyle, but that was not enough to counter the osteoporosis.

Mexican wild yam (*Dioscorea villosa*) contains a substance called diosgenin.

His meeting with Dr Ray Peat, a biochemist from Oregon, at a medical seminar in 1978 had changed his life. Years of research had convinced Dr Peat that progesterone was a very important hormone for osteoporotic post-menopausal women, for while oestrogen slowed up bone loss, the function of progesterone was to increase the formation of new bone. Furthermore, he claimed progesterone could be made from yams, soy, and indeed 5,000 different plants.

Astonished and excited by these claims, Dr Lee pursued them further, researching back to 1938 when Dr Russell Marker found plants contained fats and oils called saponins which he then discovered could be converted into 'natural' progesterone. In general, saponins are thought to be cholesterol-lowering.

During the following three years, Dr Lee monitored 100 post-menopausal white women ranging in age from 38 to 83 years (an average age of 65), using a programme of low-protein vegetable diet, modest exercise and vitamin supplementation plus a transdermal dose of progesterone.

Regular bone density tests (at six monthly or one yearly intervals) revealed:

> *Four years ago menopausal symptoms such as mood swings, forgetfulness, lack of focus, vaginal dryness and discomfort were driving me crazy. My family medical history contraindicated HRT – Mum had high blood pressure and a stroke when she was 60, I had had a breast lump and a malignant melanoma on my wrist. I read about progesterone in a health magazine, and within days, was using a progesterone cream – I think it is fantastic, it has regulated all the problems I had.*
>
> **FIONA (Cambridge)**

**TESTING TIMES**

After three months of treatment for menopausal symptoms in a double-blind placebo-controlled study using a topical product containing wild yam, researchers at the Baker Medical Research Insitute, Melbourne, Australia, found no statistical difference between placebo and active creams, even though 'mood swings' of women using the active cream actually improved in this trial. The ingredient responsible for this may well have been the geranium essential oil used in the cream.

- a reversal of osteoporosis – women actually gained bone density
- an especial increase of bone density in the lumbar region.

Not only had their bones improved, but the progesterone treatment had other benefits: the women felt better, they had less breast swelling and tenderness, their low thyroid problems improved, their high blood pressure went down and they showed a return to normal libido.

The results appeared to have potential, and before long the commercial bandwagon swung into action. Huge farms growing wild yams sprang up in Mexico, and various steroidal saponins and other plant compounds were studied. It was found that one of the richest sources for commercial use was a substance called diosgenin in the Mexican wild yam (*Dioscorea villosa*) – not to be confused with the average supermarket yam which is really a sweet potato. *Dioscorea* species have been used as remedies for at least 5,000 years for conditions ranging from rheumatoid arthritis and colic to dysmenorrhoea (difficult or painful menstruation).

It was the easy and inexpensive conversion of diosgenin into a molecule that is identical to the progesterone

hormone made by the body that paved the way for natural progesterone creams (or gels) that could be smeared on any soft skin such as a woman's tummy, inner thigh or breast.

While relief from menopausal symptoms found some support, the idea that progesterone could increase bone density was received with some scepticism.

In one way, this is heartening, given that oestrogen was once marketed as a 'wonder' drug without any knowledge of either its side-effects or long-term consequences. But in another way it is anything but heartening. There have been few clinical trials to support these claims and indeed Dr Lee's conclusion to his paper 'Osteoporosis reversal – the role of progesterone' in which he states that 'It does not require a double-blind placebo controlled experiment to conclude that progesterone is of great benefit in treating and preventing osteoporosis' hardly helped further his cause.

Whatever his humanitarian desire to help those women who could not take HRT, there is a fundamental question mark over the results of his surveys since it means there was no 'control' group not taking progesterone against whose results his sample could be compared.

This assertion that the human body could convert diosgenin in yam plants to progesterone was later refuted by Dr Lee in a book under the heading 'The Yam Scam'. He confirmed that progesterone creams do not contain any wild yam at all and that the main manufacturers use soya beans instead. Indeed Dr Lee goes on to say that:

- progesterone itself is not found in wild yams
- it is synthesized from the plant material by a number of chemical steps, which means it is not 'natural' at all
- a chemical conversion process is necessary to synthesize progesterone from diosgenins, and this can only be done by a chemist in a laboratory
- as the progesterone did not dissolve well in alcohol, and any solvents tried were highly toxic, a method was patented for dissolving it in Vitamin E.

*Within four days of starting HRT, I had 'flu-like symptoms including a raging temperature. This continued to get worse, and within ten days I was in bed unable to move. Even though she could see I was so ill, my doctor persuaded me to carry on with the HRT. But eventually enough was enough. I had read Dr John Lee's book* What your Doctor may not Tell you about the Menopause *and I knew my business partner had experimented with progesterone, so I decided to start taking natural progesterone. Within two weeks all my 'flu-like symptoms had gone.*

*We now stock progesterone at my Alternative Health Clinic and because of my experiences I am able to help customers in a similar position.*

Mo (Scotland)

The reality is that this product in the form of a cream or oil is designated a cosmetic in the USA and is available in most countries without prescription. In the UK, however, it can only be sold with a prescription although it can be obtained either by consulting a doctor in private practice or purchased by mail order or via a website company.

Great debate has raged in recent years over the issue of progesterone. Unfortunately, there is considerable dubious promotional material in respect of these products – one brochure lists 21 benefits, including 'helping endometriosis, bone building activity, restoring proper cell oxygen levels, normalizing zinc and copper levels, blood sugar and blood clotting, and facilititating thyroid hormone levels'. Furthermore, confidence in a product which is claimed to 'cure' an astonishing range of 20–30 menopausal symptoms, including anxiety, black circles under the eyes, blurred vision and constipation to water retention, sciatica, exhaustion and insomnia, is playing on the anxiety of menopausal women and offering untrialled answers to the problems associated with this time of their lives.

Other research revealed the beneficial effects of progesterone on menopause symptoms when it was tested in a small, double-blind, placebo-controlled trial: 83 per cent of the 25 women receiving 20mg of progesterone transdermally per day reported an improvement in the relief of hot flushes.

Leaving aside the question of the substantial sums of money made by commercial enterprises in its production, there are thousands of menopausal women like Fiona who are delighted with the effect of natural progesterone products on their lives.

## WHAT FORMS OF PROGESTERONE ARE AVAILABLE?

Progesterone-containing remedies come in three main forms: creams, granules and oils. The sub-lingual granules

It is claimed that the use of progesterone can cure a range of menopausal symptoms, including insomnia.

and oils, which go under the tongue, have at least three times the concentration of progesterone found in the creams. They are taken by putting a few drops of the oil or several of the granules in the mouth, and holding them there under the tongue, usually for 5–8 minutes, until they have been absorbed by the lining of the mouth.

The action of progesterone oil taken sub-lingually is much faster than that of the cream since it gets into the bloodstream straight away. The creams are effective for long-term use and maintainance.

## I AM IN MY PERI-MENOPAUSAL YEARS – HOW DO I USE THE CREAM?

Your menstrual pattern is changing at this time – probably irregular flows or missed periods – and progesterone cream can bring menstruation back to normal and keep it that way until the moment at which your menopause arrives and your periods cease altogether.

When you first take progesterone, sometimes a response called 'oestrogen rebound' can take place. This is temporary: you may experience a worsening of some of your symptoms such as breast tenderness or PMS. You might have an unexpected period because the endometrial proliferation that has built up due to the oestrogen in your body is now able to be shed thanks to sufficient progesterone being present.

The progesterone cream is used between day 12 or 13 and day 26 or 27 of your menstrual cycle. You will probably use half a jar a month during this time, but this can be adjusted according to the symptom relief.

If you stop using the cream at day 26 or 27 this usually brings on a normal period within 48 hours.

## WHERE DO I APPLY THE CREAM?

The cream can be applied to your face, tummy, breasts, back, thighs – almost anywhere on your body where there is a large area of relatively thin skin. You can apply it once or twice a day and rotate it around the different areas of your body – apply it to your tummy one day, on the thighs the next, on your breasts the next and so on.

At first, a lot of it will be absorbed into body fat. But as these fatty tissues become saturated, so successive doses of progesterone bring about an increase in blood levels and physiological effects.

### DID YOU KNOW?
At present the UK National Osteoporosis Society medical advisers do not consider there is enough valid scientific evidence to recommend the use of natural progesterone creams to prevent osteoporosis.

## HOW MUCH SHOULD I USE?

Most doctors suggest a quarter to half a teaspoon a day. You need to monitor how rapidly it is absorbed. If your symptoms increase, use more – if your symptoms decrease, use less.

## HOW LONG DO I HAVE TO USE IT TO SEE RESULTS?

This varies enormously. Some women notice relief from hot flushes almost immediately – in general, menopausal difficulties will be relieved within three months.

## WILL IT HELP VAGINAL DRYNESS?

Natural progesterone cream used on the perineum (that is the area between your vulva and anus) and intra-vaginally is generally successful is treating both vaginal dryness and vulvar dystrophy (shrinkage of the vaginal tissues). You might prefer to apply oil intra-vaginally, for example by putting a few drops of it on your finger and inserting this into your vagina.

## CAN I USE THE CREAM CONTINUOUSLY AFTER THE MENOPAUSE?

When you are post-menopausal, use it for two or three weeks a month, then discontinue for a week so that at least 5–7 days a month remain hormone-free.

## ARE THERE ANY SIDE-EFFECTS TO USING NATURAL PROGESTERONE?

No, it is not known to have any side-effects except for altering the menstrual cycle temporarily in some women, and bringing about feelings of euphoria.

Very occasionally, a post-menopausal woman will get a small period for the first month or two, then this stops permanently. Should this happen, it is a sign that the progesterone is causing your body to eliminate excess

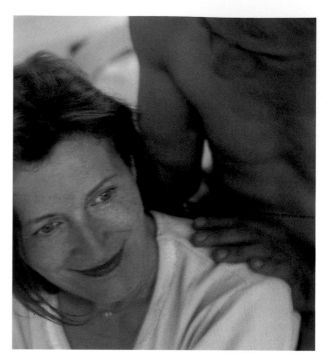

Testosterone contributes to sex drive and feelings of energy and well-being.

stored oestrogen which can trigger a shedding of the endometrium or 'breakthrough bleeding'. If any kind of breakthrough bleeding continues for more than three months, it is important to consult a doctor.

Some doctors resist prescribing natural progesterone as a part of HRT, because they feel uncomfortable about the lack of studies done on its ability to make the necessary changes in the uterus. Yet you may be someone who cannot tolerate synthetic progestogen, especially if you have a genetic tendency towards PMS, and natural progesterone may suit you better. If that is so, you will need to take higher, more frequent doses of natural progesterone than if you used a synthetic progestogen.

## Testosterone for women

In his research over the years about progesterone, Dr Lee discovered it is involved all through our bodies – from the nerves, to the brain cells, to the thyroid gland, fat metabolism, energy and muscle building. He also investigated the effects of testosterone.

Although testosterone is known as the 'male' hormone, because men have much higher levels, women also produce it. Testosterone contributes to bone and muscle strength, sex drive and feelings of energy and well-being.

In women, most testosterone is produced by the stroma, a part of the ovary, and levels are fairly consistent throughout the menstrual cycle, with perhaps a slight mid-cycle surge which increases your sex drive when you ovulate. Levels often begin to decline when women are in their late 30s or early 40s and can decrease as much as 50 per cent following the menopause. Symptoms of low testosterone levels include:

- a low sex drive, muscle weakness and loss of a feeling of well-being
- low energy, irritability, forgetfulness, crying spells, and hot flushes that do not respond to oestrogen alone
- headaches or migraines.

The role of testosterone in depression is a focus of current research, and positive effects of testosterone therapy on mood in naturally menopausal women have been reported.

## WHAT TREATMENT IS AVAILABLE?

Testosterone can be administered in the form of injection, pill or cream. Soy-based natural testosterone is available in tablets, pellets and injections, as well as gels and creams – the latter have greater absorption, produce more stable blood levels and bypass the liver.

## WILL I GROW A BEARD?

Low-dose testosterone treatment needs to be carefully monitored. It can improve sexual response, but doctors

> **DID YOU KNOW?**
> Results from the USA indicate an increase in frequency of sexual activity, orgasmic pleasure and positive well-being when transdermal testosterone was used for 12 weeks by 75 women aged from 31 to 56 with impaired sexual functioning after surgically induced menopause (hysterectomy and oophorectomy).

are often reluctant to prescribe it because of its side-effects. These include acne and virilization (enlargement of the clitoris and deepening of the voice), as well as that most feared of all – hirsuitism (excessive hair growth) – which occurs in about 5–20 per cent of women. Fortunately this effect is reversible and usually disappears when the dose is reduced.

## Summary

Hormone replacement therapy using oestrogen and progestogen offers short-term risks and benefits for the alleviation of menopausal symptoms. It also offers long-term benefits if you are at risk of certain conditions plus associated risks.

Progesterone cream appears to alleviate menopausal symptoms but as yet there is only anecdotal evidence to indicate its beneficial effects on bones, and no evidence on possible heart benefits.

A low dose of testosterone has been shown to improve libido, and is especially important if the ovaries have been surgically removed.

# 3

# Alternatives
# to HRT

# Considering the alternatives

Having read the preceding chapters, you should have a better idea about hormone replacement therapy and your own unique risks and benefits. Now you can weigh up whether or not it is right for you.

Your decision may be an easy one. For example, your menopausal symptoms are bothersome, especially your memory which is all over the place, you have always known you were at risk of osteoporosis because your mother and grandmother both suffered from it, and you now realize that HRT is also likely to protect you from Alzheimer's disease, which your father had. You do not particularly welcome the idea of continuing monthly 'bleeds' until you have had no periods for a year, but feel this is a small price to pay for the benefits of HRT.

Maybe your decision is not so clear-cut. You can cope with hot flushes in the daytime, but your night sweats are horrendous, and their impact is badly affecting both your domestic and working life. You now realize you are not at risk of osteoporosis but decide to have regular bone scans, just to be on the safe side. Your family medical history shows no evidence of either strokes, heart attacks, bowel cancer or Alzheimer's disease. In view of these factors, you decide to give HRT a try but only as a temporary measure.

Perhaps you are a woman with a disability which involves wheelchair usage. You have been feeling low and depressed, and wonder if it is hormonally based because you have had a few hot flushes over the last few weeks, your concentration is not as sharp as usual and you seem overtaken by chronic tiredness. You are reluctant to consider HRT as there is breast cancer in your family, so you decide to wait and see if any other menopausal symptoms appear. As you lead a mainly sedentary life,

you are a little concerned about being at risk of either a heart attack or stroke, so determine to increase your physiotherapy sessions and explore the possibility of hydrotherapy.

Or perhaps you believe any chemical interference in this transitional stage of your life is 'medicalizing' a normal happening. Nothing you have read in this book so far has changed your mind. Equally, you are not happy to simply 'grin and bear' your menopausal symptoms – you realize something must be done, as your moods and irritability at work have led to a tearful confrontation with colleagues. You resolve to explore alternative ways of helping yourself through this unsettling time.

## Natural alternatives

Every day, thousands of us seek help from acupuncturists, chiropractors, osteopaths, herbalists and homoeopaths as well as practitioners of other therapies such as

Alternatives to HRT may alleviate menopausal symptoms and help you to feel fitter and more relaxed.

reflexology and aromatherapy. Why should there be such interest in complementary medicine given the extraordinary achievements of orthodox medicine? For it would be hard to exaggerate the benefits that have been obtained by applying scientific principles to medicine: most bacterial infections are curable, smallpox has been wiped out worldwide and polio has ceased to be a major problem, at least in Western countries. Almost every week the media relays enthusiastic accounts of medical techniques or discoveries, such as organ transplantation, IVF and 'test-tube' babies, hip, knee and even arm replacements, cures for many cancers and gene therapy.

And yet the fact is that much of this is divorced from the daily lives of most people. For women, it is frequently menstrual disorders that badly affect their lives, often presenting as depression, headaches, backache, water retention and PMS (pre-menstrual syndrome). The end result of an (average) six-minute interview with a harassed general practitioner is most likely to be a prescription for antidepressants, painkillers, tranquillizers or sleeping tablets. Some of these are helpful in the short term – but many do not provide solutions and some even carry the potential risks of addiction and side-effects. In view of this, it is highly unlikely a therapy such as HRT could offer a universal panacea to women struggling through the 'change' from their reproductive to their post-reproductive years.

The fact that doctors are unable to guarantee the safety of prescribed drugs was all too clearly exemplified by the thalidomide tragedy in the late 1950s, when thousands of women who were prescribed a drug to counteract morning sickness in pregnancy gave birth to children with severe limb deformities. Likewise, the Opren scandal of the 1980s, and addiction to drugs such as Valium which caused its users long-term problems. Medicine has also felt the winds of change blowing through its corridors of power as a climate of accountability has entered the arena. And many patients are much more medically

literate than before, both as a direct result of medical trauma and because of the easy accessibility of information through the internet.

The combination of suspicion of drugs and disenchantment with orthodox medicine has produced fertile ground for complementary medicine.

For years, the conventional medical community has been less than welcoming of complementary medicine, and with some justification. After all, in many places anyone could rent a room, buy a leather couch, screw up a shiny brass plate outside their door, preferably with a string of impressive-sounding letters after their name – and bingo! they were in business. They could be a positive menace and danger to the potential patient – but how was the patient to know that?

The recognition of this problem eventually led many practitioners to put their houses in order: regulations, codes of ethics and competence and validation now form benchmarks for public confidence, and have paved the way for increasing collaboration with the conventional medical professions.

A poll conducted by the BBC in 1999 found that the number of people in the UK using complementary and alternative medicine had doubled over the previous six years to 21 per cent of the population. Many people claimed to have had their conditions cured or improved. Some of the commonest therapies used successfully were acupuncture, traditional Chinese medicine, medical herbalism and homoeopathy.

It would be easy to conclude that there is a powerful placebo effect at work and this attitude is encouraged by the shortage of reliable, responsible research in the field of alternative medicine in some countries, especially given that complementary medicine researchers have to compete with applicants from conventional medicine for funding.

Nevertheless, times are changing and in the USA a National Centre for Complementary and Alternative Medicine (NCCAM) was set up in 1998 to explore complementary and alternative healing practices in the context of rigorous science, train complementary and alternative researchers and disseminate the ensuing information to the public and professionals. The President's Budget for 2003 includes an estimate for over $100 million for this purpose. Unfortunately, however, they have yet to come up with research evidence into treatment of menopausal symptoms by complementary medicine. This is perhaps surprising in view of the fact that a 1997 study conducted by the North American Menopause Society reported that 30 per cent of women use acupuncture, natural oestrogen(s), herbal supplements and phyto-oestrogens to relieve their menopausal symptoms.

Personal recommendation is one way of choosing a complementary practitioner, so talk to people you know who have tried alternative therapies, and ask how they felt about the treatment they received. What did they think of the practitioner? Was the therapy being practised in clean and properly equipped premises? How much did the treatment cost, and how often did they receive it? Nowadays, reputable practitioners will include information about their membership of professional organizations in their advertisements and you should always check this out before you make an appointment.

Many complementary practitioners offer time, a sympathetic manner and therapies which are concerned with the 'whole woman'. However, this is not always the case and if, after an initial visit, you feel uncomfortable with your practitioner, trust your judgement and do not continue.

In this chapter we will explore the usefulness of complementary therapies in relation to the menopause, and you will see how many contain overlapping elements. Some, such as meditation, relaxation and yoga are self-help techniques while acupuncture requires a consultation with a practitioner.

# Acupuncture

The use of acupuncture first caught the Western imagination around 1958 when it became recognized for its effectiveness in pain control, primarily for post-operative care. Later, it was introduced as an alternative to anaesthesia during operations, first with minor procedures such as tooth extraction and later with major operations on the limbs and abdomen.

Unfortunately, this dramatic use of acupuncture led to a widespread misconception about it, as its emphasis has always been on prevention – to the Chinese, a sick man

Fine, sterile needles are inserted in the skin at relevant points. They can be left in just briefly, or be inserted for about half-an-hour, depending on the condition.

### PAIN RELIEF
Legend has it that acupuncture was first discovered by a soldier shot by an arrow who found that, when struck by a second arrow, this relieved the pain from the first.

visiting an acupuncturist is comparable to a thirsty man starting to dig a well.

Acupuncture was first used widely in China and its history is closely connected with the development of Chinese medicine in general. The theory of Chinese medicine evolved out of an era of philosophical speculation and intense consideration of the nature of life by great thinkers such as Confucius. Its four methods of diagnosis – Observing, Listening and smelling, Asking and Touching – remain as much the cornerstones of modern-day acupuncture treatment as they did in around 200BC, when a Chinese doctor, Bia Que, brought a prince out of a coma using acupuncture.

Central to the concept of acupuncture is the idea that the body is self-healing; that it is a self-rectifying whole, a network of interrelating and interacting energies. The even distribution and flow of these energies maintains health and any interruption, depletion or stagnation leads to disease. When this happens, acupuncture tries to aid the natural processes of healing, helping the body to correct itself by a realignment or redirection of energy which the Chinese call Qi (pronounced 'chee').

So what is Qi? It is often translated as breath, life-force or vitality – or simply as that which makes us alive. If there is no Qi, there is no life. Strong and energetic people have plenty of Qi; tired and depressed people lack Qi.

Along with the notion of Qi, acupuncture recognizes a subtle energy system by which Qi is circulated through the body in a network of channels or 'meridians'. The acupuncture points lie along these meridians and when the acupuncture needle is inserted, it is the Qi that is affected. In some ways the circulation of Qi is similar to the blood circulation and nervous system, although it is invisible to the eye.

The tai chi symbol shows how yin and yang are opposites, but inseparable.

Accepting this understanding of the body as an energetic and vibrating whole leads to a new approach to health and disease, for it draws together all the diverse signs and symptoms of ill-health to form a 'pattern of disharmony' which includes the mental/emotional state as much as physical problems.

## YIN AND YANG

The idea of harmony and balance form the basis of the concept of 'yin' and 'yang'. The belief that each individual is governed by the opposing but complementary forces of yin and yang is central to all Chinese thought because it is believed to affect everything in the universe.

Traditionally, yin is dark, passive, feminine, cold and negative, while yang is light, active, male, warm and positive. You and I might say that there are two opposing sides to everything, i.e happy and sad, tired and energetic, cold and hot.

The tai chi symbol on the previous page illustrates how yin and yang flow into each other, with a little yin always within yang, and a little yang always within yin. The body, mind and emotions are all subject to these influences: when the two opposing forces are in balance we feel good, but if one force dominates the other, it brings about an imbalance which can result in ill-health.

One of the main aims of the acupuncturist will be to restore and maintain your balance of yin and yang.

As you can see, acupuncture is not a system of medicine in isolation. It should be seen as one major method of treatment within a complete system that has a different perspective on health from that of orthodox Western medicine – the idea of treating a patient's headaches in one medical department, their period pains in another and their insomnia in a third would seem extraordinary to a traditional acupuncturist, since they believe there must be a common root.

Nowadays, a Westernized branch of acupuncture rejects the existence of channels or 'meridians' and believes that acupuncture works via the nervous system and that its effects can, in principle, be explained in terms of anatomy and physiology.

You will need to decide whether you are going to consult a lay practitioner (someone who may have had no formal training and possesses no accepted academic qualifications) or a doctor who is fully qualified through conventional medical training and who has undergone further training in acupuncture. Both types of practitioner are widely available.

## PINPOINTING THE PROBLEM

During your first acupuncture consultation, time will be spent asking for details about your general condition. These questions can relate to all your physical, emotional and energetic signs and symptoms and although some of

them may seem unrelated, all can help the acupuncturist to form a more complete picture of your condition.

The practitioner will also ask to see your tongue. This tongue examination is a very important source of information for the acupuncturist: the shape, colour, coating and texture of the various parts of your tongue yield information about the state of your organs. A healthy tongue should be reddish in colour with little or no fur, it should not appear swollen or contracted, neither

Your tongue can reveal a lot about the health of your organs.

Taking accurate pulse readings on each wrist is a very important part of examination by an acupuncturist.

should there be cracks on the surface or 'teeth marks' along its sides.

During the consultation, a full medical history is taken. Other important questions concern:

- eating and sleep patterns

- sensations of heat and cold, perspiration and whether this occurs during the day or night
- headaches – again when they occur and in what part of the head
- urination and defaecation, including frequency of passing urine and any tendency to either constipation or diarrhoea.

## ACUPUNCTURE AND HOT FLUSHES

Between 1995 and 1999 in Staffordshire, UK, 22 breast cancer patients, aged between 38 and 59, were referred by a consultant oncologist for acupuncture treatment of hot flushes. Analysis of this four-year study revealed that 82 per cent experienced effective relief from hot flushes and all of them recorded some reduction after completion of the course.

## SAFETY FIRST

Before undergoing any treatment, you should ask about the sterilization procedures in use at the clinic. In the UK and many other countries all registered acupuncturists are required by law to sterilize needles. Disposable needles are available if you prefer, though they will obviously be more expensive.

> *When I was 46, my periods suddenly became much heavier for six months with mid-cycle bleeding. The doctor diagnosed a fibroid and a hysterectomy was recommended. I was horrified and asked to see the acupuncturist – I am very fortunate as complementary therapists work in the same premises as my GP, so all I had to do was walk down the corridor and make an appointment. The mid-cycle bleeding stopped after two treatments and my periods normalized for about 18 months. Then the mid-cycle bleeding started again and further treatment alleviated 90 per cent of this. By now I had realized I was menopausal, so continued with acupuncture for a further year during which time my periods stopped altogether.*
>
> CAROLINE (Somerset)

## DID YOU KNOW?

The symptoms of just over 50 per cent of 300 menopausal women disappeared when treated with acupuncture at the First Hospital, Tianjin, China in 1998.

If you consult an acupuncturist for treatment of menopausal problems, you will be asked about your menstrual cycles and the menopausal symptoms experienced. You will then be asked to undress, except for your underclothes, so that the acupuncturist can examine areas of your body that are painful, to feel for heat, cold, swelling, tightness or lack of skin tone. Specific acupuncture points may be touched to see if they are painful, particularly points on your abdomen and each side of your spine.

You may be surprised that the acupuncturist takes your pulse at both wrists and in three positions, by the index, middle and ring finger. Acupuncturists believe that they can assess the balance of energy from these three positions and gain the key to your internal state. Your pulses will be checked again at intervals during treatment to monitor the energy changes.

Having gathered together all this information, the acupuncturist formulates the appropriate treatment for you. The choice of acupuncture points differs with each patient. Some points may be used repeatedly until a particular imbalance is corrected.

## TREATMENT

Acupuncture stimulates the fine network of nerves running in the skin and sometimes nerves in the deeper tissues too. These then in turn affect the central nervous system, blocking pain and altering the nervous system's control of other bodily organs. Some patients show very little sensitivity to the needles and do not feel anything when they are inserted. Others may be aware of increased sensitivity in particular areas or on particular meridians. In general, however, treatment should not be painful and when needle sensation occurs it should not last more than a few seconds. It is usually described as a 'tingling' sensation or a feeling of numbness radiating from the needle.

Treatment might be once a week to begin with, then at longer intervals as the condition responds – it depends on you and your 'pattern of disharmony'. It is demonstrably untrue to say that the results of acupuncture are 'all in the mind'. After all, treatments have been successfully carried out on very small children and animals. It is very unlikely that a cow could be hypnotized into improved health by a veterinary surgeon!

# Traditional Chinese medicine

Traditional Chinese medicine incorporates not only acupuncture, but also herbal medicines, dietary suggestions, massage and/or exercises or lifestyle recommendations. It would appear that Chinese medicinal herbs are more effective when used in conjunction with the other elements of traditional Chinese medicine.

Because of its holistic view of the body and mind, it is very specific for each patient's needs. For example, five different women coming into a clinic complaining of hot flushes, will have a variety of different accompanying signs and symptoms, no two of which are exactly alike. Therefore, each woman will receive an individually tailored treatment plan with different herbs, different acupuncture therapy and different lifestyle suggestions.

According to traditional Chinese medicine the clinical picture of hot flushes shows a deterioration in the yin of the Liver, weakness in the Blood of the Heart, and an exhaustion of the Water of the Kidney.

The deficiency of Water is countered by an excess of Fire, which endangers the control of the yin of the Liver and unleashes its yang. There are two pathological mechanisms:

- The combined effects of deficiency in the Kidney, hyperactivity in the Liver and flare-up of Heart Fire will lead to palpitation, insomnia and dizziness.
- The imbalance between the Spleen and Liver is manifested by emotional depression, irritability, loss of temper and an oppressive feeling in the chest.

Medicinal herbs are just one part of Chinese medicine.

## CONTRADICTORY EVIDENCE

Chinese herbal medicine has been used for centuries in China for treating menopausal symptoms, and some clinical trials there have shown them to be very effective.

But the outcome of a placebo-controlled trial using Chinese medicinal herbs to treat 55 menopausal women in Australia (1998–1999) found they were no more effective than placebo in reducing hot flushes and night sweats.

# Medical herbalism

There can be little doubt that plants were the first source of medicines, and the use of herbs as a source of healing remedies is inherent in all cultures in all historical times. Experience showed primitive man which particular leaves could salve a wound caused by an arrowhead, and which could be boiled to cure a fever. Evidence that the poppy was used to relieve sickness and pain has been found in some early cave dwellings, where its seed was probably used for its soporific effects.

Over the centuries, plants have been sampled for food or experimented with in an effort to find out more about their medicinal use. Who, for example, discovered that a tincture of opium from the poppy would stop children crying, or that the oil from the beans of the castor tree, in small amounts, made a reliable purgative while two or three of the beans themselves would prove fatal within a few hours? Or that the extracted oil would bring relief when applied to burns and septic wounds, as well as making a useful fuel for lamps? Yet both these plants must have been regularly used for these purposes for thousands of years: some of their seed was found in the ancient tombs of Egypt, dated 1500BC.

In primitive cultures this information was so important to the community that it was put in the care of a caste of priests/physicians. Medicine became closely associated with magic, religion and astrology. Then in 460BC the Hippocratic School attempted to separate herbal medicine from the occult and relate it to careful observation of the patient. It was Hippocrates who formulated the principle that treatment and dosage should be decided in accordance with the individual patient's requirement. This is one of the cornerstones of modern-day medical herbalism, as is the belief that the whole plant should be prescribed. Herbalists believe the whole plant is balanced by Nature in such a fashion as to make it a much safer remedy than extracted parts.

Many different herbs are used to make up the complex herbal preparations that are the mainstay of medical herbalism.

The herbal remedies of antiquity became more accessible to more people with the advent of printing during the Renaissance, but then the dawn of scientific medicine in the seventeenth century, with its emphasis on reason and experiment, challenged these doctrines. The herbalists' ancient authority was further undermined by the emergence of inorganic remedies, and herbal remedies were increasingly sidelined.

However, in every rural community since pre-history there were likely to be individuals, mostly women ('wise women') who were regarded as specialists in the art of using healing plants. They satisfied the needs of basic health care, treating injuries and illness and usually acting as midwives as well. Many of these women were tied to a larger network of 'women's culture' that handed

The beans of the castor tree have been used for their purgative properties for hundreds of years.

*I consulted a private doctor last Autumn, desperate for a way to overcome hot flushes, and her remedies have been astonishingly successful. I take Menosan drops, a tincture made from the herb sage, three times every day plus one red clover tablet once daily. Supplements and a cream have eased a few other problems I have begun or have become worse in the past two to three years.*

LINDA (London)

Nowadays, you do not need to seek out the services of a 'wise woman' for herbal remedies: you can buy them over the counter at health food outlets or via a website. On the other hand, you might choose to consult one of the 500 well-qualified medical herbalists in the UK plying their trade in a resilient herbal market worth around £65 million a year. A recent survey of the European herbal market valued the trade at 3.2 billion euro.

down the medical folklore and this culture once embraced millions of women patients. It is this folk medicine of rural communities which, blended with traditional lore of the American Indians in North America in the eighteenth and nineteenth centuries, produced the patent medicines peddled by travelling 'medicine men', 'snake doctors' and 'quacks'.

Tainted with a reputation for superstition and quackery, coupled with the influence of advances in medical science presided over by eminent doctors such as Louis Pasteur, herbal practices were again pushed into obscurity in the nineteenth and twentieth centuries. But the end of the last century saw a renewal of interest in medical herbalism, its practitioners treating those who felt uneasy about the widespread use of drugs and their side-effects.

## THE CONSULTATION

The herbalist will give you a thorough examination and will need details of your medical history and eating lifestyle. Your blood pressure will be checked and the practitioner will evaluate the overall balance of your body's systems – musculo-skeletal, nervous, cardiovascular, digestive, genito-urinary and endocrine – to discover underlying and predisposing disharmonies.

It is you as a whole person who will be treated, not simply the complaint. Thus, entirely different remedies may be prescribed to two patients apparently suffering from the same problems.

You are unlikely to need frequent consultations unless you have a condition which requires close monitoring

## HERBS COMMONLY USED FOR PERIMENOPAUSAL AND MENOPAUSAL SYMPTOMS

| Name of herb | For relief of | Recommendations |
| --- | --- | --- |
| Balm | Tension, stress reactions and depression | A tincture of 2–6ml 3 times a day, or 2–3 teaspoons of dried herb steeped in 1 cup of boiling water twice a day |
| Black Cohosh | Hot flushes, anxiety and depression | 40-200mg daily – use not to exceed six months |
| Chasteberry | Hot flushes | Prepared as a tincture, chastetree berry providesan average daily dose equal to 20mg of the crude fruit or 30-40mg of the fruit in a decoction |
| Gingko | Poor memory, mood swings, anxiety and absent-mindedness | A daily dose of 120-160mg of standardized gingko leaf extract |
| Ginseng | Fatigue, diminished work capacity and loss of concentration | 1 500mg capsule can be taken 3–6 times a day. Use not to exceed three months |
| St John's wort | Depression | 2-4g of hypericin capsule, 1-2 times a day. The equivalent may be steeped in 1 cup of boiling water for 10 minutes to gain a similar amount |
| Valerian | Insomnia and tension | 2–3g, taken 1–3 times a day, is suggested as an anti-anxiety regimen |

and regular examinations. You can simply telephone the herbalist when you need more medicine and any adjustments can be made to the remedy if necessary.

Many patients note a measurable degree of improvement within the first month of treatment, but one to two months of treatment for every year of illness may be required if the condition is chronic.

## SAFETY

It is a persistent and popular misconception that herbal medicines are totally safe and free from side-effects. However, this is far from true – after all many plants from which the remedies are made are known to be poisonous. Unfortunately, the full effects of toxic constituents of plants are difficult to assess. Under the terms of the UK Medicines Act 1968, herbal practitioners are permitted to use a few poisonous plants, such as aconite, belladonna, mandrake, hemlock and white bryony, up to statutory maximum dosages but these are not permitted for general sale. Similar regulations apply in other countries.

In 1978 Germany established Commission E to review the safety and use of over 1400 herbal drugs. The eight herbs in the table above were considered by Commission E to be effective and safe for one or more perimenopausal or menopausal complaints.

In Germany alone, 10 million prescriptions for gingko are written each year by more than 10,000 physicians.

## HERBAL PREPARATIONS

Herbal medicines come in various forms, some of which are ready for use and some of which require preparation.

Many people choose to buy ready-made preparations, but others prefer to buy the raw materials and create their own remedies. Breaking down the herb samples to a suitable size used to be the hardest work of all the processes of preparation, entailing hours of labour with a pestle and mortar, but nowadays a kitchen blender will perform many functions quite adequately.

Water or a mixture of water and ethyl alcohol is usually added to the herbs. Sometimes acetic acid (vinegar), glycerol (or glycerine) and seed oils are used. A liquid is selected which will have the best chance of dissolving the required active ingredients. 'Woody' material such as bark and roots has to be infused in hot water for a certain period.

Being natural products, herbal preparations are very variable in strength. The quantity of active ingredients will differ widely from product to product. The raw material will vary according to the climate and conditions in which it is grown, and the quality of the preparation will vary according to how it is treated and how many other ingredients are added. In addition, the dosage will depend on how you prepare it – for example, the longer teas are steeped, the stronger the dose.

## COMBINING MEDICINES

Your medical herbalist will not advise you to stop taking drugs prescribed by your doctor but will usually work together with any orthodox treatment that may be deemed necessary. Many patients want to come off their prescribed drugs and herbalists would aim to reduce or cease the need for them.

## FORMS OF HERBAL PREPARATION

| Preparation | Description |
|---|---|
| Bulk herbs | *Raw, dried plant material in jars or bins; used in teas, tinctures; powdered for capsules, tablets* |
| Oils | *External use only, some are fatal if ingested; used in aromatherapy* |
| Tablets, capsules | *Stored and transported easily* |
| Teas | *Hot-water extracts, of which there are three types:* <br> *Beverages, teas – steeped for 1–2 minutes* <br> *Infusions – steeped for 10–20 minutes* <br> *Decoctions – plant material simmered in boiling water for 10–20 minutes* |
| Tinctures | *Alcohol extracts; highly concentrated; come in small bottles with eyedropper caps; few drops usually used* |

## SAFETY CONCERNS

Much of the concern about the safety, efficacy and quality of herbal remedies may be removed following the European Union's traditional herbal medicines directive which came into force at the end of 2002. This will require manufacturers to register unlicensed products and produce them according to good pharmaceutical manufacturing practice.

## BLACK COHOSH

At present, the most effective herbal medicine for treating menopausal symptoms is an extract of black cohosh, Remifemin (known as RemiFemin in the US), which has been subjected to two clinical trials. The safety profile is positive with low toxicity, few and mild side-effects and good tolerability. Remifemin has been used in Germany since the 1950s.

## SENSIBLE MEASURES

In general, herbal medicines may have a short-term role in managing the symptoms of menopause, but they are unlikely to be useful in treating the long-term aspects, in particular the treatment and prevention of osteoporosis. Never to persist with any herbal remedy if, after a period of no more than several weeks, it is not clearly improving your condition. Most herbs do not take months to work – it is the condition which sets the pace. Always challenge a treatment if, after four weeks, you think the herbal remedy is not useful or, even if there are doubts, stop the medicine for a time and see if it is still necessary.·

## DECOCTIONS

These are made from materials such as roots, barks, nuts and seeds. Using the same proportion as for an infusion, place the mixture and water in a saucepan. Bring to the boil, then simmer for 10 minutes. Strain and drink hot.

## INFUSIONS

To make an infusion, use one teaspoon of dried herbs to one cup of boiling water; leave to infuse for 10–15 minutes, strain and drink hot. Sweeten with honey if preferred.

# Homoeopathy

Nearly two hundred years ago, an eminent and conventionally qualified German physician published the first results of a form of treatment which he had developed and used experimentally on himself and his family. His name was Samuel Hahnemann and he christened the principle of this treatment 'homoeopathy', from two Greek words – homios meaning 'like' and pathos meaning 'suffering'.

In some ways, Hahnemann was a scientist but in others he was a metaphysician or even a mystic. He believed that life was sustained by a vital force and that disease was caused by some outside influence that disturbed the smooth functioning of the vital force, thus inducing symptoms of illness. His belief was that it you could discover and remove the cause of the trouble and stimulate the vital healing force of nature then the patient would heal themselves.

It had all begun when Hahnemann decided to see what would happen if he dosed himself with quinine, a remedy used to combat malaria. He was surprised to find that he developed a fever and other symptoms associated with malaria, even though he did not have the disease. These symptoms then disappeared when he stopped taking it. But each time he dosed himself again with quinine, the symptoms recurred. Here was confirmation of Hippocrates' belief that if an individual who is suffering from an illness can be made to suffer symptoms similar to those produced by his illness, then he will be cured, and that the severity of symptoms and healing responses are dependent on the individual.

This 'like cures like' principle formed the basis of homoeopathy and is in stark contrast with conventional or 'allopathic' medicine which treats illness with an antidote rather than a similar substance. But this was not the only principle that distinguished Hahnemann's medical practice from that of his contemporaries.

Onions are just one of the substances that are used for homoeopathic remedies.

Dissatisfied with the medical practices of his day, which consisted mainly of 'bleeding' and the use of large doses of dangerous drugs, he decided to dispense smaller doses of medicine. To his surprise, he found that the more the remedy was diluted, the more active it became.

Orthodox medicine was unimpressed. This paradox – that less of a substance could be more effective – was perhaps not surprisingly unacceptable to the scientific community of the time, as well as to modern sceptics who doubt the worth of giving extremely dilute solutions of dubious substances to the sick. Nevertheless, every year 4 per cent of adults in the USA use a homoeopathic medicine, while in the UK that figure is more than double that at 8.5 per cent.

Hahnemann and his followers were ridiculed, yet they continued to experiment with all sorts of substances – derived from minerals or animal and plant products – testing them in what he termed 'provings'. Over long periods they took small doses of various reputedly poisonous or medicinal substances, carefully noting the symptoms produced. Patients who were suffering from similar symptoms were then treated with these substances with encouraging results.

An enormous amount of information was accumulated to form the main source of knowledge about homoeopathy. By the time he died in 1843, Hahnemann had done 'provings' on 99 substances. This increased to 600 more medicines by 1900 and today there are nearly 3000 substances available to homoeopaths. The materials include onion, Indian hemp, honey-bee sting venom, snake venom and spiders, as well as sand, charcoal, common salt and pencil lead. Hahnemann also advocated the use of single medicines rather than complex mixtures, reasoning that it was not possible to distinguish the effects of large numbers of drugs when they were mixed together.

There are two forms of homoeopathy in use today: one which lays great emphasis on the use of highly dilute medicines and on certain philosophical, even semi-mystical ideas about disease and its causation, and a modern form which is based on fairly orthodox notions of pharmacology and largely ignores philosophical thought. But the essence of the homoeopathic principle remains the same, i.e. it is the patient who is treated rather than the disease.

## HOMOEOPATHIC REMEDIES

A single remedy may be prescribed from a variety of sources and in a number of dilutions, such as Pulsatilla (an anemone flower), Sepia (a sea creature) or Sulphur (a mineral. The homoeopath has thousands of remedies to choose from and the process of selecting the right one is individual. Just a handful of these remedies are readily available in pharmacies and health food shops, such as:

- Lachesis for poor memory, difficulty in concentrating, anxiety and depression

## PUT TO THE TEST
A total of 657 patients received treatment for their pre- and post-menopausal complaints in a three-month study conducted in 1994 by 77 therapists in Germany.

Participants were given Mulimen, a combination homoeopathic preparation consisting of agnus castus, black cohosh, ambergris, St John's wort, common nettle, sepia, calcium, potassium and gelsenium.

Two-thirds reported continuous and definite relief from their symptoms, and even though they did not achieve complete freedom from them, all stated their intention to continue with Mulimen.

## SERIOUS ILLNESS
Responsible homoeopaths agree that many serious disorders – cancers and so on – do need treatment from orthodox practitioners.

- Pulsatilla for depression, weepiness, changeable moods and headaches
- Argentum nitricum (Arg. nit) and Salvia for hot flushes
- Graphites for irritability, difficulty in concentrating, depression, weepiness and over-excitability.

However, it can be difficult to evaluate your own situation clearly, and consulting a homoeopath for a professional opinion will result in the correctly chosen remedy in the right potency. They might be a lay practitioner (someone who may have had no formal training and possesses no accepted academic qualifications) or a doctor who is fully qualified through conventional medical training and who has undergone further training in homoeopathy.

## THE CONSULTATION

Your first homoeopathy appointment may last as long as two hours, as making the correct diagnosis is a vitally important part of the treatment. A lot will need to be known about you to build up a multi-dimensional picture of you as an individual:

- Your past health and life circumstances, the pattern of health in your family, your present condition.
- What are the particular symptoms? What makes them worse or better – warmth, cold, eating, drinking, moving about, lying down and so on?
- How do you feel about the condition? (angry, resentful, depressed?)
- What are your underlying fears, moods and anxieties?

Having gathered all the information needed, and assuming that you do not need to be referred, then the homoeopath will analyse the answers you have supplied and formulate the appropriate medicine. This can then be obtained from your pharmacist. Although they are completely different in their preparation and action, homoeopathic medicines look much like any other medicines, and are taken in the form of small pills, tablets, drops, granules, powders and liquids.

## SAFETY

Homoeopathic remedies are completely safe, non-toxic and non-addictive.

## COMBINING MEDICINES

It is perfectly safe to take antibiotics along with a homoeopathic medicine, though the side-effects from the antibiotic may complicate the symptoms picture and thus make the choice of homoeopathic treatment more difficult.

*I consulted a registered homoeopath who spent an hour-and-a-half asking me a number of questions about my general health, my current situation, major events in my life, and seemingly unrelated questions such as 'How do you feel about frogs? and thunderstorms?' She reassured me that my symptoms of irritability, mood swings, change in sexual desire, irregular and heavy bleeding, random sweating, weight gain, sleeplessness and palpitations were common when women were peri-menopausal. Having listened carefully, she then prescribed a remedy – pulsatilla.*

*The first week I took it, I experienced violent mood swings and severe irritability to the point where I almost felt out of control. I had decided to give it one more week and then give up if there was no improvement and, as if by magic, everything changed. I slept better, my periods became more regular and the bleeding lessened, my mood evened out and I became altogether more pleasant to be with, both for my family and myself.*

*I would not hesitate to recommend homoeopathy for this stage of a woman's life.*

**VICKI (Bristol)**

A number of homoeopathic substances have a very specific application in certain conditions, such as indigestion and bruising, and so they can successfully treat a large cross-section of the population. For instance, arnica ointment is very effective for healing bruises after an operation.

Some feeling of well-being is usually experienced within one week, even though the symptoms remain. However, if symptoms do not improve within two weeks of starting treatment, then an alternative medicine should be considered.

# Stress – and how to live with it comfortably

Psychosocial factors – life stress situations, depression and social isolation – have been linked to increased risk of cardiovascular disease (pages 53–59). Whatever you do in your daily life and whatever your circumstances, you will encounter stress every day. It is part of the human condition begun even before birth, for a baby can show signs of distress in its mother's womb. Stress is unavoidable, whether we are children or adults – single, divorced, married or widowed.

Stress is a catalyst for change as it provides us with excitement, stimulation and motivation. But it can accelerate to dangerous levels, and all of us need to learn ways of coping with stress.

- High levels of emotional stress increase susceptibility to illness
- Chronic stress results in a suppression of our immune systems, which in turn increases our susceptibility to illness
- Emotional stress also suppresses our immune systems and leads to hormonal imbalances.

It would be reassuring if at least our menopausal years were ones of contentment where a calmer, less frenetic pace replaced years of pressure. All too often this does not happen, because we allow ourselves to feel powerless in the face of the demands, needs and expectations of other people, frequently as a consequence of our own lack of self-esteem.

In over 20 years work as a counsellor, I have talked with hundreds of anxious midlife women about their stressful situations. One 52-year-old woman, Moira, initially described herself as being 'on a roller-coaster of confusion', and her words are echoed by many of us when we cannot see 'the wood for the trees'. This happens when our lives are so crowded that we lose sight of our own selves.

Some women find that their brains are 'on the go' all the time, and when this occurs there is a clear knock-on effect from disturbed sleep patterns. Daily living is punctuated by erratic behaviour which disrupts normal physical, mental and spiritual functioning. If this strikes a chord with you, you need to know that you can help yourself. First you need to create a quiet half an hour on your own one day with no interruptions so that you can

- identify where you are now
- reflect on and consider your options
- think about the elimination and/or better management of the stress in your life.

> I was 48 years old and had come to a crossroads in my life: I'd worked part-time as an estate agent to help my daughters through university and now wanted to do something different. I had being doing yoga for 20 years, and was encouraged to go on a teaching course in the Bahamas. It was very tough but I stuck with it and now teach three classes a week, as well as a class at the local golf club and private classes in people's homes. My dream is to have a health food restaurant with a yoga centre above it and alternative therapies on offer as well.
>
> I finally have a job that is more than merely a means to an end – I really enjoy the benefits I get from yoga and enjoy passing on those benefits to others.
>
> **JANET (London)**

Sexual intimacy may be affected during the menopausal transition, and it will need patience and goodwill to re-establish.

## From chaos to clarity

### STEP 1

You will need a large pad of paper and a pen. Divide one sheet of paper roughly into four sections and write the following words at the top of each one:

Where am I now?
Where do I want to be?
How am I going to get there?
What is stopping me?

Complete the sections with the words and thoughts that come immediately to mind – this should take about five or six minutes.

By focusing on the here-and-now, you put yourself in centre-stage, instead of the stressful situation. Maybe you have just drifted into your particular set of circumstances, with only a vague idea of what you were aiming for and put your trust in fate. Now, your concentrated effort will bring secret hopes and desires to the surface, as well as allowing for the expression of unhappy feelings.

There may not yet be total clarity, but certain words and phrases may well be thought-provoking, so much so that you find yourself scribbling down other words and thoughts on another piece of paper. You have now begun the process of putting your particular 'roller-coaster' into some sort of perspective.

### STEP 2

The first step may have stirred up all manner of emotions for you, so this next one should be undertaken only when you feel ready for it.

Read through everything you have written down and highlight stressful issues which need special attention. Group them together under the following headings:

My personal relationships
My work outside my home

Select one of these and

• explore your options
• write down the possibilities for changes, even if some of them seem far-fetched
• formulate a plan of action.

If you are unsure about the best way forward, then a session with a counsellor may help you to resolve your uncertainties.

You could also benefit from incorporating one or more of the activities and therapies covered on pages 90–103 into your life. Start by learning to relax properly using the exercises opposite.

## Learning to relax

You may think – oh, that's easy! I relax every time I come home from work, kick off my shoes and flop into a comfortable chair with my favourite tipple. And yes, some of your tension will fall away, as you relax initially in a passive, unfocused way. But not all of it, for most of us have been conditioned to believe that we must constantly be active and productive, so our minds are likely to be preoccupied with all sorts of important issues.

Many of us assume that relaxation comes naturally to us, but it does not. Setting aside time for the two exercises opposite is a simple way to start really letting go. It may well feel a bit strange at first but its effect can be both releasing and rejuvenating. These exercises can be practised while lying in bed before falling asleep or at any time when you want to achieve really deep relaxation. They feature three distinctive elements:

• a focusing on particular muscles
• tension in holding them
• relaxation.

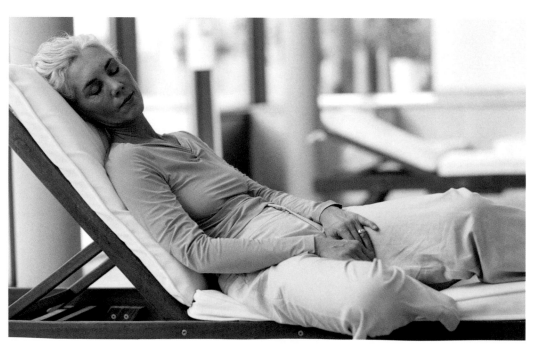

When you relax properly your entire body will be loose and totally at ease

## EXERCISE 1: A BREATHING SPACE

Your surroundings need to be warm and comfortable, and your clothes loose-fitting. If you try this exercise on the floor, then place an additional covering over it such as a large piece of foam rubber, a futon or duvet.

1. Get into your chosen position and close your eyes.
2. Focus on your breathing – feel how the air goes in and out of your lungs.
3. Feel the weight and warmth of your body – as you relax deeper into yourself, you will feel even heavier as the warmth begins to envelop you.
4. Take a deep breath, expanding your diaphragm and ribs, hold it for two seconds, then sigh, releasing all the air from your lungs. Listen to the air as it is expelled. Repeat this five or six times.

### From shoulder to shoulder

Hold each position to an even count of 5.

5. Hunch your shoulders as high as you can – hold them there – relax.
6. Tense the upper part of your arms – hold – relax.
7. Tense your complete arms – hold – relax.
8. Clench your fists – hold – relax.

### On a lower level

9. Tense your buttocks – hold – relax. Do the same with your thighs and the calf muscles in your legs.
10. Draw your feet up in the direction of your upper body, as if you are straining to see them – hold – relax.
11. Curl your toes – hold – relax.

You are now fully relaxed, and may drift off to sleep – or you can return gradually to consciousness by counting down from 10 to 1.

## EXERCISE 2: RELAXATION AND MENTAL IMAGERY

Mental imagery, also known as visualization, means forming an image in your mind, then creating a clear mental statement of what you want to happen.
Some of us are more 'visual' than others. Some people think primarily in images, wherease others tend to sense or feel things, and some people think in words. You need to operate in the sense that is most natural to you in visualizing your desired outcome.

For example, if you have high blood pressure, you could visualize the problem as little muscles in the walls of your blood vessels tightening down, so that it causes much higher pressure necessary for the blood to be driven through. Now, see the medication relaxing these little muscles in the blood vessels, your heart pumping evenly, with less resistance, and blood flowing smoothly through the vascular channels.

1. Set yourself a mental goal: for instance, the relief of repeated anxious feelings.
2. Prepare yourself with the relaxation exercises above.
3. Retreat in your mind to a special place, perhaps a tropical beach. Allow yourself to use all your senses to explore it – to feel the warm sun, smell the plants, listen to the birds, feel the salt spray on your body, the sand tickling your toes.
4. When your special place is established, put yourself into the image to achieve your goal – a relaxed mind is receptive to anything you want to give it.
5. Make a positive mental statement about yourself – 'I feel calm and in control'.
6. Drift away gradually from your special place. When you open your eyes you will feel relaxed and refreshed. Do not get up immediately as the drop in blood pressure may make you feel giddy.

# Meditation

Meditation aims to achieve both relaxation of the body and a heightened state of awareness. Regular meditation can bring greater control over restless thoughts and emotions, leading to a sense of well-being, and as a result you will be able to shut yourself off from the world and find inner peace.

It is now generally accepted that our minds can influence mechanical bodily functions and the chemical balance that ensures good health. When our minds are persistently disturbed by unhappy thoughts and feelings, such as worry, anxiety and resentment, then our energy levels become disrupted, and these then manifest as physical symptoms of illness.

Meditation can offer considerable benefits. It has been found to be effective in:

- regulating blood pressure
- stimulating blood circulation
- alleviating pain
- reducing muscular tension
- slowing down hormonal activity.

Although meditation is often associated with an ascetic, spiritual lifestyle, there is no need for you to renounce your own beliefs. It is enough to approach your meditation practice as just another element in your daily exercise routine, and take from it whatever you need – be it relief from stress, improved physical and mental health or a sustained sense of well-being.

When you first start meditating, it is important to try to establish good habits, specifically those concerning correct posture and breath control. Both of these are useful in aiding your concentration when your thoughts wander, as they will do in the early stages of meditation.

## POSTURE

Although the various postures described and illustrated on these pages are interchangeable, you could attempt all of them initially, persevering with each for a week until settling with one or two that suit you.

## Lying down

If you choose to lie down on your back, make sure you support your neck with a cushion. Let your arms hang loosely by your side and keep your legs straight. Do not cross your legs or put your hands on your body.

## Sitting

Choose a straight-backed chair to sit in so that you get support and do not cramp your diaphragm. Your feet

This is a comfortable position to relax in. Simply kneel on the floor, place a cushion behind your knees and sit down.

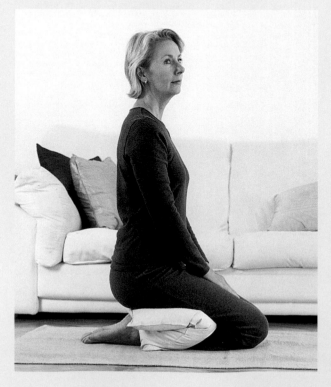

should be flat on the floor and slightly apart in line with your shoulders. Place your hands on your knees, palms down, although you may prefer to have them facing upwards in a symbolic gesture of openness.

## Classical postures

The traditional cross-legged postures that are used in yoga require a degree of suppleness you may not possess. An alternative to the classical postures is to rest on your heels with a cushion supporting your buttocks, as in the Japanese tradition.

## STARTING TO MEDITATE

Without doubt when you first learn to meditate the most difficult aspect is the quietening of the mind. Initially, you will probably find lots of other things that seem in more urgent need of your attention and you will be tempted to put off your meditation time indefinitely.

It is important to begin with simple exercises to establish good practice. This basic candle gazing meditation will help you to establish the habit of sitting still in silence and will train your mind to focus on the object of the exercise. Practise it twice a day for six days, then rest for one day before moving on to the other meditations described on page 92.

## Candle gazing

1. Place a candle in front of you so that the candle is in line with the point between your eyebrows.
2. Now gaze at the candle and observe the flicker, the candle's size and every aspect of it.
3. After 30–60 seconds, close your eyes, and keep the flame as steady as you can. At first the afterglow will fade and you will be left with nothing, so you will need to open your eyes again,

and repeat the process. You will then retain an optical image of the candle and the flicker of light in your mind.

4. When the flicker of light starts to disappear, force the image to stay. This trains your mind to concentrate hard. At first it will seem impossible to maintain the image but with continued practice it becomes easy.
5. Focus your attention on one thought, and keep breathing deeply while still focusing your mind on it.
6. Become one with the flame so that there is no space between it and you. Enjoy the sense of spaciousness and expansion.
7. When you feel ready, slowly come back to waking consciousness and open your eyes.

Learn to meditate by training your mind to focus on the flickering flame of a candle.

## OTHER MEDITATIONS

Helpful meditations in your present circumstances could include the following.

## Pain reduction

If you suffer from headaches or other pains, you may find meditation useful. A pain-reduction method involves imagining what your pain looks like:

1. Prepare yourself with the relaxation exercises on page 89.
2. Focus on your pain. What colour is it? See its colour, shape and size clearly. It may be a red ball. It may be the size of a tennis ball or a grapefruit.
3. Mentally project the ball out into space, maybe two metres away from your body.
4. Make the ball bigger, about the size of a football, then shrink it to the size of a pea. Now let it become whatever size it chooses to be.
5. Begin to change the ball's colour – make it pink, then light green.
6. Now take the green ball and put it back where you originally saw it. At this point, notice whether or not your pain has reduced.

## Getting rid of an upset

1. Get into your chosen relaxed position.
2. Close your eyes, breathe naturally and when you feel suitably relaxed, imagine that you are sitting at a desk. In front of you are pen, paper, envelope, candle, matches and a bowl filled with water.
3. Look down at the blank paper in front of you and take up the pen.
4. Now write a letter to the person who you believe has upset you, describing your feelings and explaining the situation as you understand it. It is necessary to express your feelings, as the primary purpose of this exercise is to face and free your emotions. Once you have released your anger, you will hopefully see the situation from a less

impassioned perspective, and having done so, you may well feel able to 'forgive and forget'.
5. When you have finished your letter, imagine addressing the envelope and put the letter inside.
6. Visualize lighting the candle. Hold the envelope over the flame, and when it has curled into ashes, drop it into the bowl.
7. When you feel ready, slowly come back to waking consciousness and open your eyes.

## Relationship problems

It takes two to create difficulties in any relationship, and it can be very hard to break the 'blaming' habit.

1. Get into your chosen position.
2. Close your eyes, breathe naturally and when you feel suitably relaxed, visualize the other person.
3. Soften your heart centre by meditating on compassion.
4. See the other person as a being whose human nature is as fallible as your own.
5. Draw them towards you and embrace them, while repeating the following affirmation: 'You and I are enjoying a good, positive relationship. Energy is flowing freely between us'. Then release them and watch as they fade into the distance.

Tension will be diffused and you will be able to talk matters through calmly.

Writing a letter may help you to release your anger.

# Yoga

Yoga is often seen as a mystical Eastern relaxation system which involves intricate postures that only the most supple and double-jointed of us would dare to attempt. But as many people have discovered, the movements can be very simple and beneficial whether you are nine or ninety years old, even if your joints are creaking or you are ill or disabled.

Its original practitioners some 4000 years ago in ancient India were philosophers or yogis who lived as hermits. Today, the benefits of yoga have spread internationally and it is now practised in non-religious, non-cultural-based classes all over the Western world, from local adult education classes in village halls to centres and organizations devoted exclusively to yoga. This ancient way to better health has been adopted by people of all ages and from all walks of life.

Most classes are based on hatha yoga or physical yoga – 'Ha' means the sun, which represents masculine energy, and 'Tha' means the moon, representing feminine energy.

## BASIC UNDERSTANDINGS

The three principles of hatha yoga are:
- Pranayama (breathing): This breathing technique encourages us to make full use of our lungs, balances the masculine and feminine energies within our bodies and boosts energy levels.
- Asanas (postures): These are held for as long as possible in order to build stamina as well alter the energy in our bodies.
- Dhyana (meditation).

Stretching is the best way to achieve top-to-toe fitness as well as reducing stress in your groups of muscles. In yoga exercise, stretching is an integral part of each movement. Cats are a wonderful example of stretching, and their suppleness is second to none in the animal kingdom.

Yoga is a gentle exercise system which is believed to encourage union of your body, mind and spirit and restore balance in three ways. It relaxes your muscles, improves suppleness, fitness and physical function. It relaxes your mind, and shows you how to control stress and destructive emotions. It needs to be practised regularly to have a lasting effect and is taught in classes lasting from one to two hours.

## WHAT HAPPENS IN A CLASS?

Classes vary in structure, but in a 90-minute class you would usually begin by focusing on breath control for about 10 minutes, followed by 15–20 minutes of gentle warm-up exercises. It takes time to master the postures – the teacher will reassure you about your level of achievement and encourage you not to push yourself too hard. Postures are usually performed for about 25 minutes, followed by 20 minutes of relaxation exercises. The class may end with 5–10 minutes of reflection, and advice to practise at home in a warm, quiet and well-ventilated room.

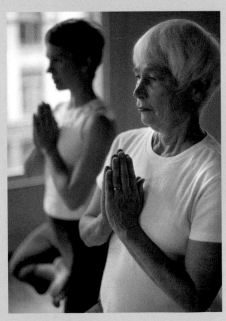

Yoga postures are usually performed for about 25 minutes in a class, followed by 20 minutes of relaxation.

# Massage

Three thousand years ago, the wealthy citizens of Greece and Rome began every day with an experience called 'the bath'. For several hours in the early morning they devoted themselves to body care. They either bathed themselves or were bathed by attendants. Intricate exercise programmes were developed to strengthen their bodies, while especially stiff muscles were rubbed with warm oils. A full body massage under the hands of skilful slaves awoke the nerves, stimulated the sluggish blood and freed the action of the joints. Finally, the entire body was rubbed with a fine oil to keep the skin elastic and supple all through the day.

The two-hour morning bath has been replaced in our advanced civilization with a five-minute experience called the shower. This is a pity because, on its most basic level, massage is therapeutic simply because it is an intensely pleasurable experience. The desire to touch and be touched is one of our strongest instincts: we touch each other to show love, to offer security, but also to make us feel better. We can exist without many things but physical contact is not one of them.

Apart from the brain, the skin is the body's most complex organ. Each square centimetre of it contains hundreds of receptors sensitive to touch, pain, pressure, heat and cold.

The basis of modern massage was developed by a Swedish gymnast turned therapist called Professor Per Henrik Ling (1776–1839). He formulated the principles of what became known as Swedish massage.

Today, massage can be found in therapy rooms, beauty salons, homes, sports clubs and hospitals.

## THE CONSULTATION

Your first appointment will normally begin with the therapist writing down details about:

- why you have come
- your current state of health
- your medical history
- details of any medication you take
- general lifestyle enquiries.

You will be asked to undress, normally in privacy, and lie on the massage table. You will not have to undress completely, you can keep on your briefs, if you wish. But even if you do strip completely, the therapist will cover you with a towel, and only uncover the parts of the body on which she or he needs to work.

The therapist might massage your back, work down your body, then ask you to turn over and work down your front, paying particular attention to knotty or tense areas. The massage should be relaxing, although you may feel pain in tense areas. You should not feel severe pain – speak out if this happens.

A full body massage can last 90 minutes, but is usually an hour. Everyone reacts differently to the treatment: you may feel relaxed, energized, slightly tired, or ache a little the next day. You might cry during the session – this is not unusual if you have been bottling up feelings.

A massage can help you to feel relaxed.

# massage for menopause

There are trigger points within the abdominal wall that, when treated, can bring relief to menopausal symptoms. Here is a massage you can ask a friend or partner to do.

**1** Place the pads of your thumbs about 7cm (3in) on either side of the navel and, using your body weight, lean in towards the navel and hold for five seconds. Repeat two or three times.

**2** Move your thumbs close together and, using the pads, work as in step 1 downwards in a straight line, from just below the navel to end level with the hips. Then work back up, finishing with your thumbs about 7cm (3in) on either side of the navel.

**3** Using very light strokes and your hands relaxed and close together, place them on the mid-abdomen, level with the navel, and stroke gently towards the groin and return. Make sure that you massage both sides of the abdomen equally.

## WHAT DIFFERENCE COULD MASSAGE MAKE TO MY STRESSFUL LIFE?

Basic massage techniques such as stroking, kneading, wringing, pummelling and knuckling, will stimulate your physical and emotional release in two ways – by a mechanical and a reflex action.

## The mechanical effects of massage

The mechanical effects are the physical results of pressing, squeezing and moving the soft tissue. This can be either relaxing or stimulating. For instance, your muscular tension can cause sluggish circulation because it forces your body's blood vessels to constrict.

Massaging the muscles frees up such tension and stimulates the circulation so that the blood flows freely, carrying oxygen and nutrients to where they are needed. It can help to normalize blood pressure, easing the pressure on arteries and veins.

Massage also stimulates the lymphatic system, encouraging it to carry waste products out of the body and defending it against infection.

## The reflex action

The reflex action is an involuntary response of one part of your body to the stimulation of another. Because your body, mind and emotions form one intricate organism, connected by energy channels and a complex nervous system with receptors in the skin, stimulus in one part of your body can affect several other parts. For example, a relaxing back massage can also ease leg pain.

## The four stages of healing

There are four stages in the healing process: relief, correction, strengthening and maintenance.

1. *Relief*
   The first few treatment sessions will relieve your pain, reduce tension and sedate stressed nerves.

They may not necessarily solve your problems, but will ease the symptoms so that you feel better.

2. *Correction*
   The therapist can now work on the underlying cause to prevent the return of the problem. Correctional work could include retuning muscles, decongesting a sluggish lymph system or freeing up fibres that are knotted or scarred.

3. *Strengthening*
   This is important if you have a badly damaged area. Massage can strengthen the surrounding tissues, enabling them to provide adequate support when your injury has healed.

4. *Maintenance*
   Your therapist may recommend a regular check-up, much as dentists do.

### THE POWER OF MASSAGE

In 1990 a study was carried out on 30 surgical patients at St Mary's Hospital, London, in connection with pain relief and insomnia. The patients were massaged on the back, face or feet and were then monitored for any physical or psychological changes. Most reported relief from pain, anxiety and muscle spasm, as well as improved sleep and general well-being. The two nurses who performed the massage also reported a better rapport with their patients.

# Reflexology

Feet and hands, two hard-working parts of the body, have always been popular sites for massage. The origins of reflexology evidently reach back to Ancient Egypt as evidenced by a wall carving in the tomb of the renowned doctor Ankmahor which shows doctors working on their patients' hands and feet. The accompanying hieroglyphics translate as the patient saying 'Don't do anything that hurts' and the doctor replying 'I shall act so you praise me', which can be seen as confirmation that this scene depicts a medical technique being used, and not a beauty treatment.

To give a reflexology treatment, a therapist mainly uses her thumb, or sometimes her finger, to apply pressure to different points to release any blockage.

Doctors in Japan, India and China developed their own methods of foot therapy, and this knowledge of Eastern therapies may have been brought to the West by adventurers such as Marco Polo who wrote that he much admired the Chinese health system.

Reflexology as we know it today was developed in the twentieth century by an American doctor, William Fitzgerald, an ear, nose and throat specialist at Boston General Hospital, using the principles enshrined in zone therapy. According to zone therapy, the body is divided into ten vertical zones, running from the tips of the toes to the top of the head and back down to the fingertips, and all the parts of the body within one zone are linked. By applying pressure to one part of the body, Dr Fitzgerald was delighted to find it was possible to relieve pain in other areas within the same zone.

Nowadays, zone therapy relies solely on the zones to determine the area to be worked, whereas reflexology takes the zones as well as the anatomical model to determine the area or areas to be worked.

## THE CONSULTATION

Your first appointment will probably last for about 90 minutes, and you will be asked about yourself and why you have come for treatment.

- Details of your medical history will be needed, including childhood illnesses, accidents or operations.
- You will need to tell the therapist if you are under the care of a doctor or receiving drug treatment for any illness or any chronic (long-term) condition.
- You will be asked how you feel about yourself and your life – your work and leisure activities, as well as your eating, drinking and lifestyle habits.

You will be asked to remove your shoes and socks or tights, and to sit down in a reclining chair or lie on a treatment couch. Your feet may be wiped with some cottonwool soaked in witch hazel, followed by an application of either cream or talcum powder, which makes it easier to carry out the treatment.

First one foot, and then the other, will be worked over by applying pressure to points on them, before giving attention to any problem areas. If you feel pain or tenderness in any area, this is an indication of a blockage or imbalance in the corresponding organ or body part. The intention is not to cause you pain, but pain is a sign of blocked energy – this can be indicated by crystalline deposits under the skin, which can feel like grains of sugar, or the reflexes can be taut or particularly spongy.

If you are relaxing in a chair, you will be able to watch the techniques used by the reflexologist. These may include the following:

- *Thumb walking*. This is done with the pad of the thumb which is pressed into the reflex points. After a few seconds, some of the pressure is released, the thumb slides along (like a caterpillar), stops and presses again.
- *Finger walking*. Similar to thumb walking, except that it is done with the side of the index finger, and using the thumb and other three fingers for support.
- *Rotating*. The thumb is pressed and rotated into the reflex point.
- *Flexing*. The toes are held in one hand while pressure is applied with the thumb of the other hand. The foot is then bent gently backwards and forwards, so that the thumb presses and releases the point in a rhythmic fashion.

No one knows exactly how reflexology works beyond the physical act of stimulating nerve endings in the feet. We know that there are 70,000 of these nerve endings on the sole of each foot which, when stimulated, can send messages along the pathways of the autonomic nervous system to all areas of the body and brain. By applying pressure to a particular point, known as a reflex point or area, the therapist can stimulate or rebalance the energy in the related zone. For example your left kidney, which is in zone 2 of the left-hand side of your body, is reflected at the same point in zone 2 of the left foot. If you have a problem in your left kidney, you might develop problems in your left eye, because the eyes and kidneys are both linked by the energy in zone 2.

## CAN IT HELP MY HOT FLUSHES?

Reflexology works well for any conditions that need to be cleared or regulated, such as menstrual irregularities, stress and fatigue and aches and pains. If you consult a relexologist for menopausal symptoms, it is likely that your feet will be worked all over, with special attention paid to the endocrine glands, and the therapist will end by pressing the solar reflex on both feet.

### PROVING A POINT

In a randomized controlled study in the USA undertaken in1993, ear, hand or foot reflexology or a placebo treatment (treating inappropriate reflex zones, too roughly or too lightly) was given to 35 women suffering from PMS. Each woman kept a symptom diary for two months before, during and after eight half-hour reflexology treatments. Thirty-nine symptoms were assessed on a four-point scale. The women given reflexology treatments showed a 46 per cent reduction in the PMS symptoms and discomfort – the placebo group had only a 25 per cent reduction.

# reflexology for menopause

A reflexology treatment can work wonders. It benefits your body's systems and also provides the relaxing benefits of a foot massage. This sequence works on the reproductive and endocrine systems, including the thyroid, to help you through the transition.

**1** First, find the thyroid reflex point, located on the top of the foot at the base of the big toe. Using your index finger, hook in and press this point for 5 seconds.

**2** Next, gently work your foot in the area between the back of the heel and the ankle bone. Gently walk all four fingers up to the ankle bone. Find the ovary point and press for a count of 5 seconds.

# Aromatherapy

If you have enjoyed a full body massage, then your pleasure may be enhanced by the addition of essential oils used by practitioners of aromatherapy. These oils are aromatic essences extracted from plants, flowers, trees, fruit, bark, grasses and seeds. About 150 essential oils have been extracted, each with its own unique scent and healing properties.

All essential oils contain antiseptic properties: some have particular ones that make them antiviral, anti-inflammatory, pain-relieving, antidepressant and expectorating. Others are stimulating, relaxing, aid digestion or have diuretic properties.

Research indicates that the scent of essential oils can exert specific therapeutic effects on our minds and emotions. The oil molecules are so small that they can be absorbed through the pores of the skin, affecting the skin itself, the bloodstream and the whole body, including the brain. Heat also helps their absorption, either through warm hands in a massage or from hot bath water.

An oil burner will release the scent of essential oils into the air, providing natural fragrance, while distributing their theraputic benefits.

## THE CONSULTATION

Your first appointment with an aromatherapist will last between one and one-and-a-half hours. As with all forms of holistic therapy, the therapist will need to know:

- about you – your medical history and why you have come
- which oils would be best to use, but also ones which should be avoided. Some oils are not safe to use if you have blood pressure problems, are epileptic or have had a recent operation
- if you are taking any medicines – or homoeopathic remedies, as strong smells can negate the effects of the latter
- what mood you are in and what kind of day you have had.

You will be asked to undress and lie down on the massage table with a towel over you (you need not undress completely if you feel uncomfortable doing so).

The therapist will leave the towel over you and move it as he or she works around your body – that way you can stay warm and also feel less exposed.

The aromatherapist might decide on a blend of oils thought to suit you or you may be asked if there are any oils of which you are particularly fond. Then, with this blend of oils, the therapist will begin your massage lasting about 30–45 minutes.

The combination of touch and the therapeutic benefits of the oils improves circulation and releases trapped energy from the muscles. The fragrance also promotes feelings of well-being. For maximum benefit you may be asked not to bath or shower for a few hours after the massage so that the oils are absorbed throroughly and completely.

Once they have done their work, the oils will leave your body in various ways: some are exhaled or excreted in urine and faeces, while others are sweated out of your system. The process can take up to six hours in a healthy person, but up to 14 hours in someone who is unhealthy or seriously overweight.

## ESSENTIAL OILS FOR MENOPAUSE

**Bergamot** is excellent for anxiety, depression and stress. It is a cleansing tonic for the uterus.

**Cypress** has a calming effect on the mind – soothing anger and frustration.

**Clary Sage** can be used for menstrual problems, depression and anxiety.

**Fennel** is good for menopausal problems such as irregular periods, pre-menstrual tension and low sexual response.

**Geranium** is useful for PMT, menopause and anxiety.

**Lavender** is good for insomnia and headaches.

You can use aromatherapy solutions at home too.

# Getting away from it all

Many women in their menopausal years feel as though they are swept along by a tide of events beyond their control without a chance for a little peaceful living. Our lives are filled with preoccupations, distractions and responsibilities, and however much we may yearn for peace, there seems little chance of making the time and space for it.

Going on retreat is a deliberate attempt to step outside ordinary life; to create a place and time of peace and quiet where distractions are at a minimum. Here is a space for you to contemplate the deepest feelings and thoughts about yourself and your relationships. Everything we feel and do is filtered through our sense of self – call it self-awareness, self-identity or consciousness, it is intrinsic to being a human.

In doing so, you may find a surprising void – an empty inner space you never knew existed. Suddenly there are no friends, children, partners, pets, television, work or the constant background of human activity. There is no gossip, no grumbling, no meetings, no decisions, no interference – you are faced with you alone. You begin to slip into a slower physical, mental and emotional gear and start to think differently – taking stock is what going on retreat is all about.

## WHO GOES ON RETREATS?

People of all ages and from all walks of life take advantage of the benefits of going on retreat – students, homemakers, grandparents, businessmen and women, millionaire celebrities and the unknown poor. Men and women of all faiths and those of none go on retreat.

You will find many different types of retreat advertised in magazines and on the internet. Most aim towards self-discovery of an experiential nature, and they can vary in duration from just a single day to a week or more.

- **Day retreats** These can be very flexible. It might be a day for silence, a day based on a theme or an activity-centred day, a time for group discussion or talks, or for lessons given in meditation technique.

- **Weekend retreats** These are often run along the following lines: you arrive on Friday evening, and, after settling your things in your room, meet the retreat leader and other guests. After supper you meet for a short talk about the weekend and are given a timetable. From that time onwards you will cease talking unless it is to the retreat leader, or during a group discussion or shared prayer. There will be time for walks, reading and just resting – simple, easy and peaceful.

- **Healing retreats** These may use prayer, meditation, chanting or the laying-on of hands.

Going on retreat means that you will have lots of time for reading, resting and quiet contemplation.

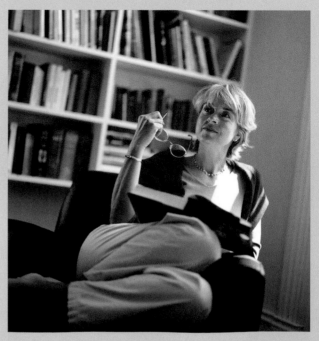

Healing may be concerned with a physical complaint or with healing the whole person in order to eliminate obstacles to personal and spiritual growth.

- **Lesbian retreats** These often have themes that bear directly on living as a lesbian within society and which link into spiritual matters.

- **Private retreats** In these you go alone as an individual. It is usually a silent time in which you find solitude in order to reflect, rest and meditate. In many monasteries and retreat houses you may arrange to take your meals in your roon or separately from others so that you can maintain this framework of silence.

- **Embroidery, calligraphy and painting retreats** Themed retreats focus on awakening personal creativity through a craft or art form. There are many other subjects as themes, such as pottery, poetry, music or gardening.

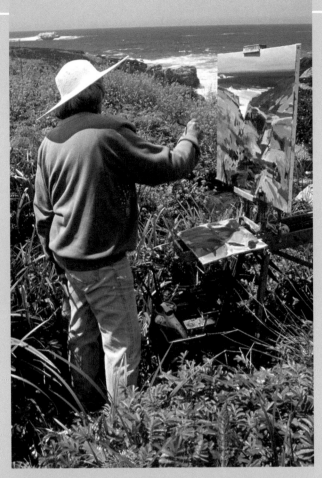

If you enjoy a craft, such as painting, then a retreat that allows you to focus on your creativity might suit you.

Having placed yourself among strangers, you may meet people you like at once, those you do not want to know better, as well as those who make a nuisance of themselves – the sort of person who has some problem and cannot help talking about it to all and sundry. Equally, you may encounter those who are certain their beliefs hold the key to life. If you do not want to listen to them, then walk away – alternatively, you might find it both charitable and instructive to really listen to what the person is saying, even if you do not believe a word of it. And you do not have to discuss any of your beliefs or feelings unless you want to do so.

Going on retreat is about refreshing yourself, relaxing and taking a journey into your deeper self. Reassessment about your life and relationships and values can happen. And why not? When have you ever had time to do this?

## BEFORE YOU BOOK...

If you have a disability, you will need to double-check the facilities before booking as many retreat centres and guest accommodation have not yet been updated to the national standard set for the disabled.

# 4

# Seeds of change

# Your diet and the menopause

The previous two chapters have demonstrated the variety of options open to you when considering HRT and its natural alternatives.

You may be convinced by the women in Chapter 2 who have spoken about their zest for living, happier feelings and renewed energy levels when taking HRT, both for menopausal symptoms and as a long-term therapy – and this is what you want for yourself. The simplicity of this treatment is especially appealing as you juggle the working/domestic elements of a busy life. But you have also given more thought to these pressures, and realize you run a real risk of 'burnout' unless you take time out for yourself. Reading about all the benefits of yoga has inspired you to find out about classes held in your area.

Perhaps you are booked into hospital for a hysterectomy and oophorectomy (removal of ovaries), and you are unable to take HRT afterwards because of your family

Cycling can be fun when away from crowded cities, and is excellent exercise, whatever your age.

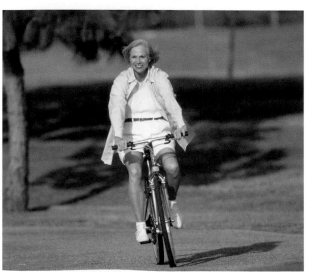

history of breast cancer. Your doctor has strongly emphasized the need for low-dosage HRT post-operatively, and that regular mammograms will monitor your situation. You now realize there is a possible option in taking the SERM raloxifene (see page 49), and perhaps combining it with progesterone cream to counteract the abrupt loss of important hormones following the operation plus a herbal/homoeopathic remedy if your menopausal symptoms re-surface.

On the other hand, you may be delighted to find that relief of your menopausal symptoms is possible when using herbal or homoeopathic remedies, as you consider HRT unnecessary for this transitory stage in your life. As your vagina is sore and painful during sexual intimacy you decide to discuss this with your doctor and ask for a prescription for a vaginal ring.

However, there is another important consideration which affects all of us whatever our ages: it is what might be termed 'food fitness' and in this chapter we shall explore what this means.

## A question of balance

Perhaps you think you have maintained a healthy eating lifestyle while cooking for your family, but you are alarmed to discover that a dress you bought a couple of years ago doesn't fit – is this middle-age spread?

Taking stock of your eating and drinking habits now will stand you in good stead for the rest of your life. This does not mean giving up food and drink you enjoy, rather

'Tell me what you eat: I will tell you what you are'   (Jean-Anthelme Brillat-Savarin, 1825)

Using a steamer to cook food preserves all the vitamins which are often lost in conventional cooking.

recognizing how you can benefit by introducing exciting new perspectives to it as well as modifying some of the less helpful ingredients.

As a child some 60 years ago, the food and drink I consumed was basic, nutritious, wholesome – and predictable. I recall wholemeal bread, meat and two veg, rice pudding and lots of milk. Today, the impact of foreign trade and travel is reflected in the food we buy: pizzas, curries and rice as well as vast ranges of pastas, sauces, cereals, cheeses, fish, meat and exotic fruits and vegetables – all stimulate our taste buds and empty our wallets. Theoretically, Western society is now better fed than ever before. The reality is that many of us live in a 'toxic food environment' of cheap fatty food, pervasive food advertising and sedentary lives.

Added to which, however self-assured and confident we are about our choice of sustenance, almost every week

dire warnings appear in the media about the dangers of meat/coffee etc., yet contradictory statements extolling their virtues are as likely to hit the headlines in the future. So how do we sort out fact from fiction?

## Back to basics

Your body needed nutrients to maintain your physical, mental and emotional well-being from when you were a foetus in your mother's womb. As you developed from babyhood, essential nutrients determined your growth, and your food is made up of the following three elements:

- Carbohydrates
- Protein
- Fats

### CARBOHYDRATES

Carbohydrates are your body's main source of energy for all its functions. They exist in all vegetables, fruits, starches and grains and, in its purest form, in refined sugar.

There are two types of carbohydrates – complex and simple. Complex carbohydrates give a slow release of energy because it takes time for our digestive tracts to break them down into the simplest substances that our bodies can use. Simple carbohydrates are best avoided where possible: they will make your blood sugar curve rise steeply as a lot of sugar is pumped quickly into your system. The curve is then forced to drop off quickly, so that after a couple of hours, your energy levels will plummet and you will feel hungry again.

### Complex carbohydrates

- Grains – wheat, rye, oats, rice, barley and maize
- Beans – lentils, kidney beans, chickpeas, etc.
- Vegetables
- Fibre in grains, beans and vegetables

## Simple carbohydrates

- Fruit, honey, white and brown sugar, and glucose in high energy drinks.

You may be surprised to see fruit described as a 'simple' carbohydrate. Fruit (and honey) contain fructose (also called fruit sugar) which is a simple sugar, but the fibre content of the fruit is a complex carbohydrate that slows the digestion rate. Fructose is fine when taken in whole fruits, like apples and pears, but not when used in the refined form of powdered white fructose.

## PROTEINS

Proteins are found in their largest concentrations in animal foods such as meat, fish, poultry, eggs and cheese, vegetables, foods such as nuts and seeds, and in high-protein legumes such as beans.

## FATS

There is more confusion about dietary fat than almost anything else. It is seen as the villain of our eating habits, responsible for weight gain and its ensuing sluggish metabolism. We have all read about low-fat diets and

### PROSTAGLANDINS
Beneficial prostaglandins (hormone-like regulating substances) are made by our bodies from omega-3 oils. These prostaglandins are particularly useful at the time of menopause as they help lower blood pressure and decrease sodium (salt) and water retention.

no-fat diets – indeed, many of us have tried them. Sorting out fact from fiction about the nature of fats will help you determine how much you should increase/decrease its inclusion in your 'food fitness'.

Basically, there are two types of fat – saturated and unsaturated:

## Saturated fat

This is found in meat, dairy products like cheese, ice-cream, milk and tropical oils like palm kernel oil and coconut. If you eat too many foods full of saturated fats they will do their best to lay themselves down as fat stores – hence the connection between fat intake and hardening of the arteries (see page 54).

Olives and olive oil are an excellent source of omega-3 essential fatty acids.

Oily fish, such as mackerel, contain oils that can help prevent the onset of heart disease.

## Unsaturated fat

This is a group of fats which includes those called essential fatty acids (EFAs). These are essential for our health: they are a vital component of every human cell and our bodies need them to insulate our nerve cells, keep our skin and arteries supple, balance our hormones and keep us warm.

Unsaturated fat comes in two forms: mono-unsaturates, like olive oil, and poly-unsaturates, found in corn, sunflower seeds and peanuts. Within this group there is a further division into:

## Omega-3 fatty acids

The most important of these is alpha-linolenic acid, found in fish oils and linseed oil, walnuts, pumpkin seeds and dark green vegetables.

## Omega-6 fatty acids

The most important of these is linolenic acid, found in unrefined safflower, corn, sesame and sunflower oils.

Our bodies can make all the fat needed for our daily metabolic processes except for these two essential fatty acids: Omega-3 and Omega-6.

The essential fatty acid (EFA) linolenic acid is converted to gamma-linolenic acid (GLA) which is found in evening primrose oil. Great claims have been made for the powers of evening primrose oil, especially for its success in treating PMS and it is popularly believed to suppress menopausal flushing. Your intake of essential fat can be improved by including the following:

- Cold-pressed unrefined vegetable oils such as sesame and sunflower oil for salad dressing
- Extra-virgin olive oil for cooking
- Oily fish such as mackerel, sardines, etc.
- Nuts (almonds, pecans, brazils, etc.) and seeds (sesame, pumpkin, sunflower, etc.)
- Tahini (creamed sesame seeds) for sauces and dressings
- Butter in moderation for spreading or cooking.

# On the go all the time

Pause for a moment and look at your body – it is relaxed and still. What you cannot see is that the inside of it is an energy machine, never resting, always metabolically alive. This machine powers its operations mainly through the use of a basic sugar molecule called glucose. Your body must have glucose, and even under conditions of starvation, it will continue to obtain it as long as there is anything in your body which it can convert into glucose. All of the food you eat is broken down into glucose via the digestive system, and is absorbed through the wall of the intestines into the bloodstream. Once that happens, you then have a high level of glucose in your blood, and your blood sugar levels are said to be high.

## AS THE BLOOD GLUCOSE RISES

As your blood sugar levels go up, which they do after eating simple carbohydrates, such as a bar of chocolate, your body has to make an instant decision – how much of that pure energy should be used for immediate needs and how much should be stored for future requirements?

The instrument for this decision is the hormone insulin, produced by the pancreas, because insulin governs the chemistry of sugar in the body. A rise of sugar in the blood elicits a swift response from insulin, which quickly converts part of this glucose to glycogen, a starch which can be stored in muscles and the liver and which can be made readily available for energy use.

But what happens if all these glycogen areas are full, and there is still more glucose in the blood than is needed that moment? In this case insulin stimulates the conversion of the excess glucose to fat molecules called triglycerides: these are part of the overall profile of fats in the body and are frequently elevated in people with heart disease and diabetes.

## THE ROLLER-COASTER GLUCOSE RIDE

Sadly, all those delicious sweet cakes, chocolates and cookies that make our taste buds drool are full of ingredients that are refined. This means that the flour, for example, has been finely processed, and the outer bran of the seed discarded. Most of the fibre is also removed. Fibre absorbs water and contributes to the growth of beneficial bacteria in your gut. This process makes a bulky stool, providing exercise for your bowel and keeping your intestine in healthy working order.

When you eat foods high in such refined ingredients, then digestion is very fast and glucose enters your body rapidly, causing your blood sugar levels to rise steeply. In addition, any food or drink which contains a stimulant, such as coffee, tea, alcohol or chocolate, causes a sharp and rapid rise in blood glucose, which may make you feel temporarily more energetic. However, the effect is short-lived. Blood sugar levels soon slump again because simple carbohydrates are unable to maintain them.

When this happens, we feel tired and put on the kettle to make a cup of tea or coffee, then eat a chocolate biscuit – hey presto! – we are revived, full of energy once more.

But this boost has caused our blood sugar level to go up rapidly, so repeating the cycle of blood sugar swings. Over time, this roller-coaster stimulation exhausts the pancreas, so that it becomes unable to produce sufficient insulin to regulate blood sugar levels. The result is that too much glucose stays in the blood, instead of being converted into energy or body fat.

If we have not eaten for three hours, our blood glucose will drop to quite a low level so we again look for the quick boost. At the same time our adrenal glands will make our livers produce more glucose. The combination of these two causes high levels of glucose in our blood which again calls on the pancreas to over-produce insulin in order to reduce the glucose levels. The roller-coaster ride starts all over again and our adrenal glands become exhausted because of repeated stimulation.

## WHY SHOULD THIS MATTER WHEN I AM MENOPAUSAL?

There are many reasons why it is important to avoid the roller-coaster effect on blood sugar levels described above. Maintaining a steady blood sugar level can make a huge difference to how you feel emotionally and physically before, during and after the menopause. Its imbalance puts you at risk of diabetes. And it is especially important during the menopausal years because of the effect on the adrenal glands. As described earlier (page 11), these glands convert androstenadione into oestrone which will be the main source of oestrogen after the menopause. They also produce a hormone called dehydroepiandrosterone (DHEA) which has been linked to anti-ageing. It is therefore crucial that the adrenal glands are working to their optimum.

Since the maintenance of steady blood sugar levels is such an important factor during the menopause then it clearly makes sense to modify or change your intake of food and drink accordingly. This will be of benefit not only at this time but also for the rest of your life.

## Looking East

In Japan, China and Indonesia women so rarely experience hot flushes that their languages do not have words for this menopausal symptom. On the other hand, eight out of ten American women reportedly experience what are termed 'power surges' or 'hot flashes'.

The explanation for this discrepancy, experts say, can be found in diet. The typical diet in the Far East is high in soy and, in Japan, low in processed and refined foods and high in mineral-rich seaweed and fresh fish oils. Not only do Japanese women eating a traditional diet have fewer incidences of hot flushes – they also have lower rates of breast cancer.

The rate of reported menopausal symptoms is also lower in other Asian women, although this could be attributed to a culture that raises its women to 'Never complain, never explain'. It has been noted that when Asian women move to the West and assume a Western diet, then they rapidly develop the diseases encountered there.

## RECENT CHINESE STUDY

The China Diet Study began gathering information on the lifestyles of 6,500 adults in 1983. One hundred people from each of the 65 provinces comprising China answered 367 questions about their diets, lives and bodies. This ten-year study is the most comprehensive study ever done on the eating habits of Chinese people.

It was an exacting, labour-intensive study, initially financed by the US National Cancer Institute, that could probably not have been done anywhere except China. Nowhere else is there a genetically similar population with such great regional differences in

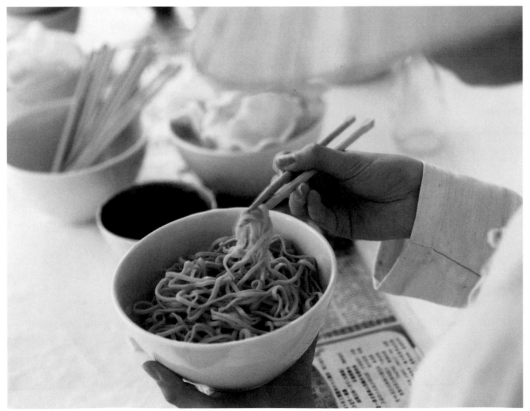

Far Eastern food is often low in processed and refined ingredients.

disease rates, dietary habits and environmental exposures. And nowhere else could researchers afford to hire hundreds of trained workers to collect blood and urine samples and spend three days in each household gathering exact information on what and how much people ate, then analysing the food samples for nutrient content.

It was money well spent, for it has turned out to be a very important study – unique and well done, and challenges much of dietary dogma.

Highlights of this 920 page study show that:

Legumes, such as lentils, contain phyto-oestrogens.

- Chinese people consume 20 per cent more calories than Americans do, but Americans are 25 per cent heavier. This is because the Chinese eat three times the amount of starch and only one-third the amount of fat. This is a more important factor than exercise.
- Cholesterol levels in China are much lower than in the USA. The Chinese average is 127mg/dL, compared with 212mg/dL in the US.

Japanese diets are often high in mineral-rich seaweed.

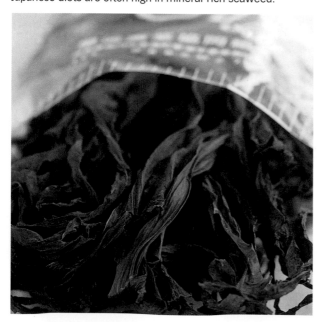

- Protein intake in China is one-third less than in the USA – 64g (2¼oz) per person per day, compared with 100g (3½oz).
- While Chinese women eat only half the calcium that American women eat, osteoporosis is uncommon in China. Most Chinese people eat no dairy products at all and obtain their calcium from plant foods.
- In China, mortality rates from colon cancer are lowest where cholesterol levels are lowest.
- For every heart attack in China, there are 16 in the USA.
- Female cancers relate to diet. A childhood diet high in protein, fat, calcium and calories promotes rapid growth and early onset of menstruation. This increases a woman's risk for developing cancer of the reproductive organs and the breast. Chinese women rarely get these cancers and they begin menstruating 3–6 years later than American women.
- The Chinese diet is three times richer in fibre than the American diet, resulting in relatively low rates of colon cancer in China.
- Iron-deficiency anaemia is rare in China, though their diet is mainly plant food and they eat less meat than in the West. The average Chinese

adult consumes twice the iron the average American does, but the vast majority of it comes from plants.

- While Chinese women eat only half the calcium that American women eat, osteoporosis is uncommon in China. Most Chinese people eat no dairy products at all and obtain their calcium from plant sources.

# Soy far, so good

Some plants contain substances that, when eaten, can affect hormone status. These substances are called phyto-oestrogens.

Perhaps the most famous example of this is the soya bean. Soya beans contain phyto-oestrogens known as isoflavones, which make up about 75 per cent of the soya protein. In the human gut, enzymes convert these into compounds that can have an oestrogenic action, even though they are not hormones. Although the potencies are considerably weaker than the oestrogen produced by the ovaries (estradiol), they appear to mimic and modulate oestrogens and can help to stabilize hormone fluctuations. Depending on the tissue and the concentration, phyto-oestrogens either act as hormones or they inhibit the actions of natural hormones. In this way they may do a similar job to tamoxifen (the breast cancer drug), which binds onto oestrogen receptors and inhibits breast cancer growth.

Foods that contain phyto-oestrogens include:

- Wholegrains (such as wheat, corn and oats)
- Legumes (such as chickpeas, mung beans, lentils and peas)
- Garlic
- Linseed
- Sunflower and pumpkin seeds,
- Almonds, cashews and peanuts
- Radishes
- Potatoes
- Fennel
- Celery
- Sprouting beans (such as alfalfa)
- Parsley
- Green tea
- Papaya
- Rhubarb
- Apples.

However, it is the soy products like tofu (soya bean curd), tempeh, miso, tamari (wheat-free soy sauce made in the traditional way), natto, okara and yuba, as well as soya milk and soya protein powder, which are the simplest ways to incorporate phyto-ocstrogens into your meals.

A recommended daily dose of 45g (1½oz) of soy protein has been found to reduce hot flushes by 40 per cent.

# A slice of good fortune

Nearly 20 years ago, a woman living in Yorkshire, England, made a momentous decision, little knowing what would develop from it. Linda Kearns had been on hormone replacement therapy for 13 years following a hysterectomy and oophorectomy (removal of ovaries) but had never really felt 100 per cent. She always felt tired and a little under the weather. Following a breast cancer scare, she decided enough was enough and stopped taking HRT. Her hot flushes and night sweats re-appeared overnight.

She began reading up about alternative remedies, and discovered she could replace the HRT using foods rich in phyto-oestrogens. The problem was that some natural seeds and grains on their own are rather unappetising, so Linda set about creating a tasty cake.

## A SLICE A DAY TO KEEP FLUSHES AWAY

Within three weeks of starting to eat the resulting cake, her menopausal symptoms disappeared and she was bursting with energy. She now eats two slices of her cake every day at breakfast and after her evening meal.

When word got out, she found herself inundated with a request for the recipe (see right). Today, upwards of 2000 of these cakes (available in raisin, cherry and cranberry), are baked every day at a Yorkshire bakery.

About 100g (4oz) a day (or a third of a 300g (11oz) cake) is usually adequate to deliver sufficient phyto-oestrogens to relieve menopausal symptoms. A 100g (4oz) slice looks generous, but it does not have to be eaten all at once. And you don't need to worry about the sugar and fat content: there are no added fats other than those naturally occurring in the various seeds, and no added sugar.

## Recipe for the Linda Kearns Cake

### Ingredients

| | |
|---|---|
| 100g (4oz) soya flour | 2 pieces of stem ginger, |
| 100g (4oz) wholewheat | finely chopped |
| flour | 200g (8oz) raisins |
| 100g (4oz) porridge oats | Approx 750ml (1¼pt) soya |
| 100g (4oz) linseeds | milk |
| 50g (2oz) sunflower seeds | 1 tablespoon malt extract |
| 50g (2oz) pumpkin seeds | ½ teaspoon nutmeg |
| 50g (2oz) sesame seeds | ½ teaspoon cinnamon |
| 50g (2oz) flaked almonds | ½ teaspoon ground ginger |

Place the dry ingredients in a large bowl and mix thoroughly, then add the soya milk and malt extract. Mix well and leave to soak for about half-an-hour. (If the mixture is too stiff, add more soya milk.) Spoon into two loaf tins lined with greaseproof paper and oil. Bake in the oven gas mark 5/190°C/375°F for about 1¼ hours or until cooked through. (Test for this with a skewer.) Turn out and leave to cool.

The cake is delicious with butter or spread. Ideally, eat a slice a day.

**Note** *The cake is not artificial HRT. It is a cake containing only the ingredients listed, which themselves contain natural plant phyto-oestrogens.*

# Good health off the shelf

If you read glossy magazines, listen to commercial radio or watch TV, or if you explore the plethora of health websites on the Internet, you will know that there is a thriving industry devoted to the promotion of vitamin and mineral supplements. These are aimed at people concerned about a variety of conditions and increasingly, combinations of vitamins and minerals are being marketed for specific groups of people, such as menopausal women.

Adverts often feature an amazing display of attractively presented pills, potions and packets, bristling with complicated neo-scientific data on the labels – so how do you decide which, if any of them, will improve or maintain your health?

First of all, you need to know what the various vitamins and minerals do in the human body.

## VITAMINS

- **Vitamin A** maintains your healthy skin, eyes, bones, hair and teeth.
- **Vitamin D** assists in the absorption and metabolism of calcium and phosphorus for strong bones and teeth.
- **Vitamin E** helps protect your red blood cells, circulation and heart. As an antioxidant, vitamin E helps to protect cell membranes, fats and vitamin A from destructive oxidation.
- **Vitamin K** is needed for proper clotting of your blood and is vital for bone formation.
- **Vitamin C** (ascorbic acid) is important for maintenance of your bones, teeth, collagen (which makes up 90 per cent of our bone matrix) and blood vessels. We neither manufacture nor store our own vitamin C, so

**RED BLOOD CELLS**

Red cells float in the blood and are the means by which oxygen reaches all parts of the body. They contain a protein, haemoglobin, which has a special ability to grab oxygen molecules as the cells circulate through the lungs and then release it wherever it is needed in the tissues. Iron is an essential constituent of haemoglobin, and anaemia is the result of lack of haemoglobin.

Pernicious anaemia results not from lack of iron but from lack of Vitamin $B_{12}$.

we need to make sure that we obtain adequate amounts during the day.

Four of the B group vitamins – $B_1$, $B_2$, $B_3$ and $B_6$ – release energy from the food we eat, as well as performing other functions.

- **Vitamin $B_1$** (Thiamine) is needed for a normal appetite and for the functioning of a healthy nervous system.
- **Vitamin $B_2$** (Riboflavin) is necessary for healthy skin and eyes.
- **Vitamin $B_3$** (Niacin) helps to maintain the skin, nervous system and proper mental functioning.
- **Vitamin $B_6$** plays a role in protein and fat metabolism and is essential for the function of red blood cells.
- **Vitamin $B_5$** (Panthothenic acid) fights infections and strengthens the immune system.
- **Vitamin $B_{12}$** (Cobalamin) prevents pernicious anaemia and is necessary for a healthy nervous system.
- **Vitamin $B_{17}$** (Amygdalin) is purported to control cancer.

## MINERALS

- **Calcium** protects and builds bones and teeth and aids blood clotting.
- **Chromium** breaks down sugar for use in the body and helps to regulate blood pressure.
- **Iron** aids growth, promotes the immune system and is essential for metabolism and production of haemoglobin.
- **Manganese** is needed for normal bone structure and is important for both the hormone production of the thyroid gland and for digestion.
- **Magnesium** is extremely important for the health of your bones, equally if not more important than calcium (see box, opposite). You need twice as much magnesium as calcium if the biochemistry of your bone formation is to run smoothly.
- **Phosphorus** maintains healthy, strong bones and teeth and is necessary for muscle and nerve function.
- **Potassium** regulates your body's water balance, aids muscle function and helps to dispose of the body's waste.

Spinach is a rich source of iron and vitamin K.

### MARVELLOUS MAGNESIUM

Sixty per cent of your body's magnesium stores are contained in your bones, particular the trabecular bone of your wrist, thighs and vertebrae. Magnesium is vital in metabolizing calcium and vitamin C, and helps to convert vitamin D to the active form necessary to ensure proper calcium absorption.

- **Selenium** is a trace element that occurs naturally in the soil, foods and your body. It is a potent antioxidant, preventing or slowing down ageing, vital to activate thyroid hormones and keep your liver functioning healthily.
- **Sulphur** helps to fight bacterial infection, aids your liver and forms part of tissue-building amino acids.
- **Sodium** (salt) is essential for normal growth and helps muscles and nerve function. It is, however, excessive in most people's diets.
- **Zinc** is present in small amounts as a component of insulin and is required for blood sugar control, and needed for hearing and proper taste. It is also important for wound healing, and assists the activity of vitamin D in promoting the absorption of calcium.

From the chart on page 118–121, you will be able to check and see exactly what vitamins and minerals feature in your current diet. Once you have done this, you might realize that you do not eat enough foods containing vitamins $B_1$ or $B_{12}$, or minerals such as magnesium or potassium, so increasing them with a supplement could be the answer. Equally, you may not like drinking milk, or eat much in the way of dairy products, so this chart will show you other foods from which you can gain calcium.

## CALCIUM SUPPLEMENTS

If you decide to buy a calcium supplement, look very carefully at the label. Calcium carbonate is the cheapest and most widely marketed calcium supplement – it is otherwise known as chalk. Be aware that calcium carbonate is an inorganic mineral; it is mined from the ground and is not present in this particular form in any plant or animal. It can increase your risk of kidney stones and is not even particularly well absorbed into the body's system. On the other hand, calcium citrate is absorbed well. The following test will show you if the supplement you are taking is being absorbed: place your supplement in a glass of warm vinegar for 30 minutes, stirring every few minutes. The warm vinegar roughly represents the conditions found in your gut. If the supplement does not dissolve after 30 minutes, try another type.

## Sensible supplements

Supplements are regularly dismissed by nutritionists as being unnecessary, but they are the answer if you have neither the time nor inclination to prepare nutritious food, or you are reassured by taking a tablet which contains a specified daily requirement. There is growing evidence that they can have a beneficial effect on menopausal symptoms, especially the following:

- Lambert's Gynovite Plus – multivitamins and minerals for women during and after the menopause (recommended by the UK Women's Nutritional Advisory Service).
- BioCare Isoflavone Complex (fermented soy and vitamins B6 and E) (Biocare products are available in Europe as well as Singapore, South Africa, Israel and Oman).
- BioCare Phytosterol Complex (natural source of plant sterols).
- Solgar Earth Source (suitable for vegetarians). Solgar has spent several years employing rabbinical supervision to obtain kosher

certification – look for the KOF-K symbol on these products. This supplement is manufactured in the USA and sold in 20 countries worldwide.

## Fatty acids

If you decide to take an appropriate vitamin and mineral preparation, the next most important nutritional group for long-range supplementation is the essential fatty acids. As mentioned earlier in this chapter, they are a vital component of every human cell and your body needs them to

- insulate your nerve cells
- keep your skin and arteries supple
- balance your hormones, and
- keep you warm.

Linseeds provide a source of omega3 fatty acids. Biocare's linseed oil (flaxseed oil) is manufactured in either capsule form or lemon-flavoured powder in 500mg or 1000mg.

Linseeds can be bought as seeds or as oil.

# Food fitness

Try to buy high-quality food from good sources and eat:

- Fruits and vegetables – abundantly
- Wholegrains and cereals – moderately
- Beans, peas and lentils – often
- Fats and concentrates (i.e. foods that are high in protein, fat or sugar) – sparingly.

The following foods are all rich sources of minerals and vitamins.

### FRUIT

Apples *vitamins A, $B_1$, $B_2$, $B_3$, $B_{17}$, C, D and E, iron and manganese*

Apricots *sodium, zinc and vitamin $B_{17}$*

Avocado *manganese, vitamins B, C and E*

Bananas *potassium, chromium, vitamins B and C*

Blackberries *vitamins B, C and E*

Cherries *vitamins B and C*

Cranberries *vitamin C*

Damsons *vitamins B and E*

Dates *sodium, vitamin B*

Figs *sodium, sulphur, vitamins B and C*

Grapefruit *potassium, phosphorus, vitamins B and C*

Grapes *Iron, vitamins B, C and E*

Gooseberries *vitamins B, C and E*

Guavas *vitamin C*

Kiwi fruit *vitamin C*

Lemon *vitamins B and C*

Loganberries *vitamins B and C*

Mangoes *vitamins B and C*

Melons *vitamin C*

Nectarines *zinc, vitamin $B_{17}$*

Olives *sodium*

Oranges *magnesium, vitamin C*

Papaya *vitamins A, B₁, B₃, B₅*

Passion fruit *vitamins B and C*

Peaches *manganese, vitamins B and C*

Pineapple *vitamin C*

Plums *iron, vitamins B₁₇ and C*

Quince *iron, vitamins B and C*

Raspberries *sodium, sulphur, vitamins B, C and E*

Rhubarb *vitamins B, C and E*

Strawberries *sodium, sulphur, vitamins B and C*

Tomatoes *potassium, vitamins B, C and E*

Tangerines *vitamins B and C*

Ugli fruit (a citrus fruit indigenous to Jamaica, a cross between a grapefruit and a tangerine) *potassium, phosphorus, vitamin C and magnesium*

## VEGETABLES

Artichokes *potassium, vitamins A, B and C*

Asparagus *potassium, vitamins A, B, C and E*

Aubergines *magnesium and phosphorus, vitamin B*

Beans *vitamin B₁₂*

Beetroot *vVitamin C*

Broccoli *selenium, vitamin E*

Brussels sprouts *sulphur, vitamin C*

Carrots *sulphur, vitamin A, B and C*

Cauliflower *potassium, vitamins B, C and E*

Courgette *vitamins B and E*

Garlic *sulphur, vitamins A, B₁, B₂, B₃, B₅ and C*

Kale *calcium, phosphorus, potassium, sulphur, vitamin A*

Leafy green vegetables *iron, vitamins B₂, C*

Mushrooms *vitamins C and E*
Okra (an African plant, also called gumbo) *magnesium, sulphur, vitamins B and C*
Onions *selenium, sulphur, vitamins B₃ and C*
Parsley *vitamins A, B₃, B₅, and E*
Parsnips *sulphur, vitamins B, C and E*
Peas *calcium, vitamins B and C*
Peppers *vitamin C*
Plantain *vitamins B and C*
Potatoes *calcium, chromium, sulphur, vitamin C*
Pumpkin *iron, zinc, vitamins B and C*
Radishes *potassium, vitamin C*
Red cabbage *magnesium, vitamins B and C*
Savoy cabbage *vitamins B, C and E*
Spinach *calcium, iron chromium, vitamins B, E and K*
Spring cabbage *vitamins B and C*
Spring onions *vitamin C*
Squash *iron, phosphorus*

Sweetcorn *vitamins B and E*
Watercress *vitamins B₃, C and D*
White cabbage *vitamins B and C*
Yams (sweet potatoes) *vitamins A, B and C*

## DAIRY FOOD

Butter *enjoy occasionally*
Cream *resist!*
Cheese *vitamin B₂, enjoy in moderation, see the Calcium chart*
Eggs *sodium, sulphur (egg yolk), zinc, vitamins B₂, B₁₂ and E*
Milk *vitamins B₁₂, D and calcium*
Yogurt *vitamins A, B, D and E*

## MEAT, FISH AND SHELLFISH

Bacon *buy the best! Grill rather than fry*
Herring *vitamins B₂ and D*
Oysters *zinc, vitamin B*
Quahog (an edible clam) *phosphorus, selenium*

Salmon *calcium, vitamins $B_2$ and D*
Tuna *phosphorus, selenium, vitamins $B_2$ and D*

## BEANS

Chickpeas *vitamins C and E*
Soya beans *calcium, potassium*
Soya flour *vitamin B*

## SEEDS

Pumpkin seeds *iron, zinc, vitamins B and C*
Sesame seeds *calcium, phosphorus, vitamin $B_1$*
Sunflower seeds *vitamin $B_1$*

## NUTS

Almonds *calcium, magnesium, vitamins $B_2$ and E*
Barcelonas *vitamins B and C*
Brazils *iron, phosphorus, vitamins B and E*
Cashews *magnesium, vitamins B and E*
Chestnuts *potassium, vitamins B and C*
Coconut *sulphur, vitamins B, C and E*
Hazel *vitamins B and E*
Peanuts *vitamin $B_1$ and E*
Pecan *vitamins B and C*
Pine *vitamin B*
Pistachio *vitamin B*
Walnuts *iron, magnesium, vitamins B, C and E*

## GRAINS AND CEREALS

### BREAD

The staff of life. (Take care with some white breads as they may contain sugar or dextrose and/or flourimprovers – the latter is fine if it states 'Ascorbic acid' on the label as this is a form of Vitamin C.)

Chapatis *vitamin B*
Rye bread *vitamins A, $B_1$, $B_2$, $B_3$, $B_5$, $B_{12}$ and E, and manganese*
Wholemeal bread *chromium and manganese*

### BREAKFAST CEREALS

(Read the label to check sugar content.)
Bran *selenium, phosphorus, iron, vitamin $B_1$*
Oats *magnesium, sodium, vitamin $B_1$*
Rice *iron, magnesium, phosphorus, vitamin $B_1$*
Wheatgerm *zinc, magnesium, vitamins $B_1$ and E*

## BEVERAGES

Champagne *enjoy!*
Cocoa *zinc, vitamins B and E*
Coffee *reduce*
Tea *manganese, vitamins B and C*
Water *Drink 8 glasses of water a day*
Wine *vitamin B is in red wine excellent for your heart!*

## SWEET TREATS AND SAVOURY SNACKS

Biscuits *avoid, they are usually full of refined sugar*
Cakes *resist!*
Chocolate *special treat only!*
Crisps *vitamins B, C and E*
Danish pastries *resist!*
Honey *calcium*
Ice cream *calcium*
Jam *vitamin C*
Peanut butter *vitamins B, C and E*
Sugar *Refined white has no vitamins, demerara and muscavado contain vitamin B*

# 5

# Get moving!

# Exercise

The advantages of regular physical exercise are numerous and well-documented. Exercise allows us to burn fat more efficiently, and it boosts our metabolism so that we continue to burn off calories at a faster rate even after we have stopped exercising, thereby helping to control body weight.

Exercise can have a powerful all-round effect on your health. Regular exercise helps to keep the bowels working efficiently, which gets rid of waste products your body does not need.

In addition, it

- improves the function of the immune and lymph systems, and the ability of the body to keep blood sugar levels in balance
- maintains bone density
- maintains muscle mass
- increases metabolism, burning calories and fat
- reduces stress
- alleviates many menopausal symptoms, such as hot flushes

Exercising with a friend can be an extra motivation.

- helps former smokers stay off cigarettes
- boosts the immune system, lessening vulnerability to colds and 'flu
- helps maintain flexibility and joint movement as you age.

## A healthy heart

Regular exercise is vital to keep your heart healthy. Research consistently shows that it keeps arteries flexible and reduces cholesterol levels.

Aerobic exercise – which speeds up your heart rate – is considered ideal for a healthy heart, so aim for 30 minutes of aerobic activity such as swimming, brisk walking, running and cycling at least three times a week.

Start gently and build up gradually. Mild breathlessness is normal and healthy.

### COUNT THE CALORIES

How many calories do you burn off doing everyday activities? This is how much you can use up in 20 minutes:

| Activity | Calories burned |
|---|---|
| Ironing | 20 |
| Housework | 60 |
| Digging the garden | 100 |
| Walking upstairs | 120 |
| Running upstairs | 200 |

## KEEPING UP THE PRESSURE

Physical activity can help to keep your blood pressure low, and an hour of brisk walking five times a week is recommended for maximum benefit.

# Build bones and muscles

Your bones and muscles need weight-bearing exercise to boost bone density. Such as high-impact activities include:

- skipping
- aerobics
- tennis
- running
- gentle weight-training.

# Exercise your mind

Your mental health will also benefit from regular exercise. Physical activity releases 'feel-good' endorphins, which boost your mood and help you to relax.

Swimming and jogging can also help to calm your mind, while your mood will be lifted by steps accompanied by music – dancing is guaranteed to 'banish the blues' of a difficult menopause (see page 138).

## ENDORPHINS
Endorphins are chemicals secreted by the brain which help us to feel happier, more alert and more calm.

# Getting motivated

Going to a gym or health fitness centre may suit you and your lifestyle – but it may not. Many of us are put off by the membership fees and the need to buy the right gear, as well as worrying about our exposure in front of strangers. It is easy to feel intimidated or uncomfortable, and you will soon lose your motivation if you don't enjoy the experience.

But many gyms and leisure centres offer a huge range of possibilities – from salsa and belly dancing to kickboxing and rockclimbing – so it is worth taking the time to investigate what is available.

Swimming is a fun way to exercise.

# leg swing

This exercise will improve your flexibility and circulation. Use a cushion if you find your joints are uncomfortable when kneeling on the floor.

**1** Kneel on all fours. You can do this exercise with or without small hand weights. If you choose to use them, place one in the bend of your right knee. Lift you lower leg slightly to keep the weight in place.

**2** Lift the bent knee until it is level with your spine and your right foot is pointing up to the ceiling.

**3** Swing your bent leg down and through until your knee is under your chest. Return it to the starting position and lower to the ground. Repeat the exercise using the other leg.

# kneeling hand walk

This exercise places much needed pressure on your hand and arm joints and bones. Make sure that your spine is kept straight by not letting your head hang.

**1** Kneel down on all fours, keeping your back straight.

**2** Keeping your knees and feet still, slowly walk your hands forward until your arms are carrying much of your weight. Be sure to keep your spine straight.

**3** Now walk your hands out to the side. This will greatly increase the strength of the bones in your arms. Then walk your hands back in the reverse pattern until you are kneeling comfortably, balanced on all fours again. Repeat this a few times and then stand up.

# Posturing with purpose

In childhood we have a naturally relaxed posture, but as we mature our bodies start to reflect the strains of life. It is easy to get into the habit of slouching in a squashy armchair or of sitting hunched in front of a computer screen without taking a break. Some jobs necessitate standing for long periods or performing repetitive actions. All these occupations can place undue stress on specific parts of our bodies.

Every day we acquire incorrect posture without noticing that it is happening, and this in turn filters through to other physical functions and depletes our energy.

Other postural problems can have an emotional basis – people who carry an emotional burden can often be seen to literally carry it on their shoulders.

One condition which can be rectified by particular exercises is kyphosis. This curvature of the top of the spine is sometimes associated with osteoporosis, and is therefore frequently seen in post-menopausal women.

If kyphosis is becoming a problem for you, you may find it helpful to make the Pilates system part of your daily routine. This exercise system was formulated by Joseph Pilates, a German gymnast, skier, boxer, wrestler and physical fitness trainer, and is based on the premise that our physical movements most benefit our health when they are conscious actions serving our will. So whether we are walking, sitting, turning or stretching, we should always direct our movements, clear in our minds as to exactly what we are doing and how advantageous it will be to us.

Pilates is different from other forms of exercise primarily because of its holistic approach and its combined training of mind and body to achieve correct postural alignment. Its key elements are

- lengthening short muscles and strengthening weak muscles
- improving the quality of movement
- focusing on the core postural muscles to stabilize the body
- working to place the breath correctly
- controlling even the smallest movements
- understanding and improving good body mechanics
- mental relaxation.

BAD POSTURE          GOOD POSTURE

Good posture is not just about having a straight back. It lends balance to our limbs, allowing movements such as walking to be performed more smoothly. We all have our own unique way of walking and an awareness of your body's posture can add balance and control to what are otherwise unconscious movements, such as standing, sitting and lying.

## Standing

If you watch people standing – say at a bus stop, on a station platform or queuing at a check-out – you will notice how often they simply do not know what to do with their bodies.

They put the weight on one leg, bending the other – then shift their weight to the other leg. There is an attempt to stand up straight, but knees get locked and the pelvis is pushed forward, creating an exaggerated hollow in the lower spine. And as for arms – we do not know what to do with them! They get folded across our bodies, or hands are clasped behind our backs, or we place our hands on our hips. It is as if we have no sense of gravity within our bodies. If we can find it, it will hold us in a position of balance and ease.

### HOW TO STAND

- Stand with your feet hip-width apart.
- Make sure that both your legs are facing forward.
- Your legs need to be straight but your knees should not be locked back into the joint.
- Allow your arms to rest naturally at your sides, falling over the middle of your hips.
- Feel your weight being supported by the middle of each foot.
- Do not rock back, allowing the heels to take your weight, or place your weight on the balls of your feet.

The strains of life can be reflected in poor posture.

Once you have achieved this way of resting with your muscles relaxed and your balance centred you will find that you tire less easily, feel taller and are more relaxed in your environment.

## Sitting

Like standing, sitting is something we often do not do very well. We sit balanced on one hip bone, then we shift to the other. We cross our legs or sit with one leg underneath us. We wriggle around in our seats, trying to find a position that is comfortable. When we eventually do find a comfortable position, it does not seem to last long.

We try to find external solutions to this, such as lumbar supports on chairs or car seats. The trouble with these is that they are not suitable for most of us – they are too low down to give support where it is needed. Instead, they tend to push the lumbar spine forward, and this in turn can push the abdominal muscles and the internal organs forward.

You should be able to place both feet flat when you sit down.

### CHOOSING A CHAIR

When looking for a chair which will properly support the back and allow you to adopt a good sitting posture, you need to check out the following:

- You should be able to sit comfortably with your whole thigh supported by the seat of the chair.
- You should be able to place both feet flat on the floor comfortably.
- The back support should be as high as your shoulder blades – the backs of many office chairs are either lower or higher than this.

Remember to sit with your weight evenly distributed, your knees slightly apart in order to support the weight, and your feet together, underneath your knees.

## Lying down

We spend approximately a third of each day lying down. Again, we do not give much thought to this, we just do it, and as we are sleeping for much of this time, we are unaware of our position.

Lying down should be our ultimate position of rest, but still we manage to contort ourselves in various ways that put strain on our muscles and limit our blood circulation. How often have you woken up with stiff muscles and a sore back? Sleeping on your stomach will not support your spine, as it often gets twisted if one leg is bent up when you are in this position. To breathe properly while lying on your stomach, your head has to be turned to one side. This not only twists the neck but can also trap nerves in it, leading to feelings of numbness or 'pins and needles' during sleep or waking.

The best positions for sleeping are either on your back or side. If you have a lower-back problem, it can be helpful to sleep with a pillow between your knees.

# Wake-up time!

How often do you wake up and instinctively feel like a good stretch even before you put a foot out of bed? Quite often your whole body moves into that stretch, elongating your back, your arms and your legs, but without you consciously willing them. You might even yawn while you do it – another reflex action. Stretching your body like this feels pleasurable, but how good is it for you?

Stretching helps to lengthen your muscles and to relax them. If we think of our muscles as having the same qualities as elastic bands, it is easy to understand the aim of doing stretches. Too much tension tightens our

muscles, and makes us feel tired and depressed. Relieving the muscle tension by stretching brings back elasticity and aids muscle/joint harmonization.

Tight muscles cause a number of problems, and as the muscles are interconnected, an injury or condition may not arise in the area of tightness, but instead in an area connected to it. For instance, lower back injuries can result from tight hamstring muscles at the back of the knees. Tight hamstrings restrict mobility and result in your lower back also being tight. Very tight hamstrings pull on your pelvis, creating postural problems.

Stretching your muscles should feel comfortably uncomfortable. The sensation should be one of stretching, not one of tearing. Take care! If you experience a hot, shooting pain while stretching then stop the exercise immediately, otherwise you are likely to cause damage.

While you sleep you will change your position many times.

# hamstring stretch

The hamstrings are the two tendons at the rear of the hollows of your knees. Tendons are constructed of tough, inelastic fibrous tissue that connects a muscle with its bony attachment. This pilates exercise will help you to stretch them.

**1** Place your buttocks on the edge of a desk or the arm of a sofa, just enough to support your pelvis. Place the heel of one foot on a low stool in front of you. Make sure that the stool is close enough for you not to have to stretch your leg out to reach it. Turn your foot outwards to stretch your buttock and hamstring muscles.

**2** Next, turn your foot inwards to stretch the inner part of your hamstring.

# shoulder stretch

This is a pilates exercise that will help you to stretch your shoulders. Repeat this exercise 3–6 times.

**1** Kneel with a cushion between your knees and calves. Squeeze the cushion and clasp your hands behind your back at the level of your buttocks. Breathe in, pull up your pelvic floor and pull in your stomach muscles.

**2** Breathe out, pull your shoulders back and squeeze your shoulder blades together.

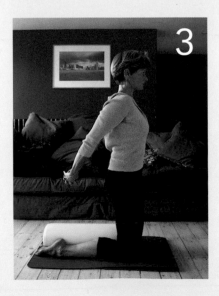

**3** Stretch your clasped hands away from your buttocks. Hold the position for 3 breaths.

# neck stretch

The aim of this pilates exercise is to stretch and relax your neck muscles. Repeat each of these steps 1–3 times.

**1** Sit on the edge of a chair or bed. Tuck your chin in towards your chest. Allow yourself to melt like an ice cube from your chest and stomach muscles, letting the spine drop forwards. Hold the position for 10–30 long slow breaths.

**2** Drop your right ear towards your right shoulder as far as it is comfortable. Hold for 10–30 long slow breaths.

**3** Now drop your left ear towards your left shoulder as far as it is comfortable. Hold for 10–30 long slow breaths.

# cat stretch

This exericise will help to increase your spinal articulation.
Repeat this exercise 3–6 times.

**1** Start on your hands and knees, making sure that your hands are beneath your shoulders and that your hips are above your knees. Make sure that your back is flat and that your head and neck are in alignment with your back, parallel to the floor. Breathe in, sensing the breath coming in between your shoulder blades. Pull up your pelvic floor and pull in your stomach muscles.

**2** Breathing out, curl your tailbone underneath you, push into your hands and lift your breastbone, tucking your chin and then your head underneath. Hold this position and breathe in. Breathe out and lower yourself back into the starting position (step 1) by reversing the sequence, bringing your head back up to its position parallel with the floor, followed by your chin and tailbone.

# Get fit without the fuss!

There are lots of ways in which you can introduce more exercise into your lifestyle without making big changes.

- If your workplace is close to your home, you could get up a little earlier, leave your car at home and walk to work – you will be doing your bit for the environment that way as well!
- If you have a longer journey, get off the subway, bus or train two stops earlier. A brisk 20 minute walk each day is excellent for getting your heart pumping, and you will feel refreshed and energized when you start work.
- Housework and gardening can both help you work up a sweat: push the vacuum that much harder, rake the lawn more energetically, and stretch up with that feather duster – it all makes a difference!

- Get into the habit of taking a lunchtime stroll. Just walking to the sandwich shop will boost your fitness levels, and help you avoid that post-lunchtime energy slump.
- If you work at home, it is theoretically easier to take a break, but in practice you need to discipline yourself to build in time for exercise. It helps to have a dog – dogs are always pleased for an opportunity to go walkies!
- Alternatively, you could exercise at home in front of an exercise video.
- If sexual intimacy is part of your life, then vigorous sex can be a great form of exercise, boosting your heart rate, increasing your lung capacity and giving your muscles a workout. However, sex may be the last thing on your mind until your menopausal symptoms are under control, and an understanding partner can make all the difference.
- If you are spending the day shopping, try walking between shopping areas, rather than jumping on the bus or in the car – carrying bags is a good way to combine a walk with weight-bearing exercise.

Walking to work, or walking for part of your journey, is an easy way to increase the amount of exercise you do each day.

If you don't want to join an exercise class, try visiting your local gym and using their exercise machines.

- When you are shopping in a department store, take the stairs instead of the lift or escalator. Climbing stairs helps tone your leg muscles and raises your heart rate.
- Stretch, skip and jog for 5–10 minutes while you are watching the TV or listening to music.

## Some commonsense precautions when starting to exercise

- If you are over 50 and have health risk factors or have been extremely inactive, see your doctor before starting an exercise programme.
- Exercise must be regular. A weekend blitz – where your usual sedentary self suddenly leaps into six hours of tennis – is more dangerous than helpful.
- Stop if you feel short of breath, a muscle strain, joint pain, or numbness and tingling, especially in your chest and arms.
- Use the right shoes. Exercise has become shoe-specific, with walking shoes for walking, step shoes for step aerobics, and many kinds of running and aerobic dance shoes. You may be tempted to use the same pair for every activity, but an investment in proper shoes is essential – for the sake of your feet!
- Do not overlook the importance of sleep. If you are suffering menopausal night sweats, then your sleeping pattern will be totally out of kilter. It is important to try to catch up on sleep as and when you are able to.
- If you need some instruction, get it. Books and videos can give you an idea on how to get started, but if you want to go past the basics, join a class.
- Drink a glass of water before and after exercising. Do not rely on thirst as an indicator of how much water you need – if you are thirsty, you are already water-depleted.

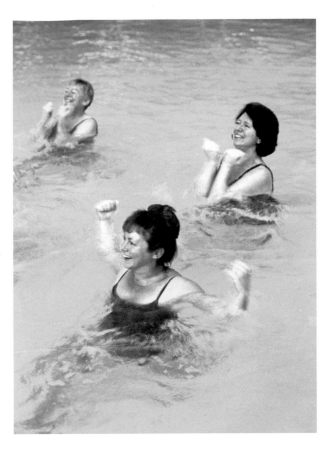

Find out about local exercise classes. You may be surprised at the amount of activities you can join in.

- Sports such as golf and tennis are fun and a great way to socialize, but because the nature of the sports require you to constantly start and stop, they rarely keep your heart rate consistently high enough to qualify as aerobic exercise.
- If you want to build your stamina and maintain a healthy heart, then choose continuous-movement activities such as walking, swimming or aerobic dance classes.

### SHOULD I EXERCISE WHEN I FEEL ILL?

If you have a headache, stuffy nose or you are sneezing, try exercising for 10 minutes, then evaluate how you feel. If you feel fine, continue. But if you have a chesty cough, stomach pain or muscle strain it's best to skip your exercise session a day or two.

If you don't want to join your local gym, why not try dancing lessons instead.

## Let's dance!

You may have holidayed abroad and returned with glowing memories of cultures in which dance is a vital part of life.

And what a choice we have worldwide! Where once social dancing was restricted to the traditional ballroom, nowadays clubs offering instruction in flamenco, lambada, line-dancing and breakaway swing (jiving plus a few solo moves) have sprung up all over the place, with salsa and Argentine tango particularly on the rise.

Dancing is an instinctive celebration of our physical state of life – we do it when we feel good, and we feel good when we do it. For it puts us in touch with ourselves and with others – the touch of another person confirms we are real, we are alive.

An evening's dancing as is as good a form of exercise as a three-hour hike. Dancing:

- releases energy and emotion
- pumps blood up our legs, so it's good for our hearts
- keeps our brains tuned
- promotes supple posture and relaxation
- encourages self-confidence and a sense of achievement as we master a new skill
- gives us the opportunity to get up close and personal to a range of partners, in a setting where ability and enthusiasm transcend age, gender and class.

Whatever your choice of exercise – enjoy it! If the 'feel-good' factor is missing, then try something different.

*Nobody cares if you can't dance well. Just get up and dance. Great dancers are not great because of their technique, they are great because of their passion.*

MARTHA GRAHAM,
US dancer and teacher (1895–1991)

# Bibliography

**Chapter 1**

Booth, M., Beral, V. and Smith, P.
*Risk factors for ovarian cancer: a
case control study.*
*British Journal of Cancer 60,*
May 1989.

Celso-Ramon Garcia, and Berg
Cutler, Winnifred. *Preservation of
the ovary: a reevaluation. Fertility
and Sterility.*
*The American Fertility Society 42(4),*
October 1984.

Ford, G. *Listening to your
Hormones.*
*Prima,* 1996.

Green, A. et al. *Tubal sterilisation,
hysterectomy and decreased risk
of ovarian cancer.*
*International Journal of Cancer 71,*
1997, pp. 948–951.

Loft, A. et al. *Incidence of ovarian
cancer after hysterectomy: a
nationwide controlled follow-up.*
*British Journal of Obstetrics and
Gynaecology 104(11),* 1997,
pp. 1296–1301.

Mason, A. *Health and Hormones.*
*Penguin Books,* 1960.

Melville, A. *Natural Hormone
Health.*
*Thorsons,* 1990.

Sellman, S. *Hormone Heresy.*
*Getwell International,* 2000.

Teaff, N. and Wiley, K.
*Perimenopause – preparing for
the change.*
*Prima,* 1999.

Yaegashi, N. et al. *Incidence of
ovarian cancer in women with prior
hysterectomy in Japan.*
*Gynaecology and Oncology 68(3),*
1998, pp. 244–246.

**Chapter 2**

Beckham, N. *The wild yam scam
when not to believe the
unbelievable.*
*Townsend Letter for Doctors and
Patients,* Feb–March 2002.

Clark, J. *Hysterectomy and the
Alternatives.*
*Virago, 1993;* Vermilion, 2000.

Coney, S. *The Menopause Industry.*
*Spinifex Press,* Australia, 1991.

Day, L. et al. *Randomised factorial
trials of falls prevention among
older people living in their own
homes.*
*British Medical Journal 325,* 2002,
p.128.

Dibba, B. and Prentice, A. et al.
*Bone metabolism.*
*American Journal of Clinical Nutrition
71,* 2000, pp. 544–549.

DiSaia, P.J. and Brewster, W.R.
*Hormone Replacement Therapy
for survivors of breast and
endometrial cancer.*
*Current Oncology Reports 4,* 2002,
pp. 152–158.

Duvernoy, C.S. and Mosca, L.
*Hormone replacement therapy
trials: an update.*
*Current Atherosclerosis Reports 4,*
2002, pp. 156–160.

Felson, T. et al. *The effect of
postmenopausal estrogen therapy
on bone density in elderly women.*
*New England Journal of Medicine
329,* 1993, pp. 1141–1149.

Fogelman, I. *Screening for
osteoporosis.*
*British Medical Journal 391,* 1999,
pp. 1148–1149.

Gennazini, A.R. *Hormone
Replacement Therapy and
Cardiovascular Disease: the current
status of research and practice.*
*Parthenon,* 2002.

Grodstein, F. et al. *Postmenopausal
hormone use and risk for colorectal
cancer and adenoma.*
*Annals of Internal Medicine 128,*
1998, pp. 705–712.

Hulley, S., Grady, D., Bush, T. et al. *Randomised trial of estrogen and progesterone for secondary prevention of coronary heart disease in post-menopausal women.* *Journal of the American Medical Association 280,* 1998, pp. 605–613.

Kenton, L. *Passage to Power.* *Vermilion,* 1996.

Key, T. et al. *Dietary habits and mortality in 11000 vegetarians and health-conscious people: results of a 17 year follow up.* *British Medical Journal 313,* 1996, pp. 775–779

Kivipelto, M. et al. *Midlife vascular risk factors and Alzheimer's disease in later life.* *British Medical Journal 332:* 2001, pp. 1447–1451.

Lee J.R. *Is natural progesterone the missing link in osteoporosis prevention and treatment?* *Medical Hypotheses 35,* 1991, pp. 314–318.

Lee JR. *Osteoporosis reversal – the role of progesterone.* *International Clinical Nutrition Review 10(3),* July 1990.

Michels, K.B. *The contribution of the environment (especially diet) to breast cancer risk.* *Breast Cancer Research 4,* 2002, pp. 58–61.

Morrisey, D. et al. *Management of the climacteric. Postgraduate Medicine 108(1),* 2000.

Mosca, L., Collins, P., et al. *Hormone replacement therapy and cardiovascular disease. A Statement for healthcare professionals from the American Heart Association.* *Circulation 104,* 2001, p. 499.

Murphy, S., et al. *Milk consumption and bone mineral density in middle aged and elderly women.* *British Medical Journal 308,* 1994, pp. 939–941.

Prentice, A. *Osteoporosis.* *Proceedings of the Nutrition Society 56,* 1997, pp. 357–367.

Purdie, D. and Crawford, I. *Management of the symptomatic menopause.* *Pharmaceutical Journal 263(7070),* 1999, pp. 750–753.

Ridley, M. Genome – *The autobiography of a species in 23 chapters.* *Fourth Estate,* 1999.

Schairer, C. et al. *Estrogen-progestegen hormone replacement therapy associated with greater increase in breast cancer risk than therapy with estrogen alone.* *Journal of the American Medical Association 283,* 2000, pp. 485–491.

Shifren, J. et al. *Transdermal testosterone treatment in women with impaired sexual function after oophorectomy.* *New England Journal of Medicine 343,* 2000, pp. 682–688.

Thomas, T. *A role for estrogen in the primary prevention of Alzheimer's disease.* *Climacteric 4,* 2001, pp. 102–109.

## Chapter 3

Bradford, N. *The Hamlyn Encyclopaedia of Complementary Health.* *Hamlyn,* 2000.

Eden, J. *Herbal medicines for menopause: do they work and are they safe?* *Medical Journal of Australia 174,* 2001, pp. 63–64.

Feder, G. and Katz, T. *Randomised controlled trials for homoeopathy.* *British Medical Journal 324,* 2002, pp. 498–499 (Editorial).

Glenville, M. *Natural Alternatives to HRT.* *Kyle Cathie,* 1997.

Israel, D. and Youngkin, E. *Herbal therapies for perimenopausal and menopausal complaints.* *Pharmacotherapy 17(5),* 1997, pp. 970–984.

Oleson, T. and Flocco, W. Randomized controlled study of premenstrual symptoms treated with ear, hand and foot reflexology. *American Jounral of Obstetrics and Gynecology. 82(6),* December 1993.

Roland, P. *How to Meditate.* Hamlyn, 2000.

Simonton, O.C. *Getting Well Again.* Bantam Books 1978.

Whiteaker, S. *The Good Retreat Guide.* Rider, 2001.

Wiegnand, M. *A gentle alternative in the therapy of perimenopausal symptoms.* Biology Therapy X11(1), 1994.

**Chapter 4**

Atkins, R. *Dr Atkins New Diet Revolution.* Vermilion, 1992.

Cooke, B. *Nutritional supplements in herbal practice.* European Journal of Herbal Medicine 3, 1997.

Davis, S. *Phytoestrogen therapy for menopausal symptoms?* British Medical Journal 323, 2001, pp. 354–355.

Diehl, Hans. *Huge diet study indicts fat and meat.* Lifeline Health Letter September-October 1990 (discussion of the China Diet Study).

Husband, A. *Phytoestrogens and menopause.* British Medical Journal 32A, 2002, pp. 52.

Mayo Clinic. *Soy and hot flashes: more heat than substance?* www.MayoClinic.org, 2000.

Mervyn, L. *The Dictionary of Vitamins.* Thorsons, 1984.

Norman, J. *Aromatic Herbs.* Dorling Kindersley, 1989.

Oliwenstein, L. *That certain age.* Vegetarian Times July 1999.

Savarin-Brillat, J.A. *The Physiology of Taste.* Penguin, 1970 (first published 1825).

**Chapter 5**

Blount, T. and McKenzie, E. *Pilates System.* Hamlyn, 2001.

# Index

## A

acupuncture, 72–6
adrenal glands, 11, 110
adrenaline, 12
aerobic exercise, 124
ageing process, 19, 24, 44
alternative medicines
    see complementary medicines
Alzheimer's disease, 25, 41–2
amenorrhoea, 13, 52
anaemia, 115
androgens, 11
angina, 53
argentum nitricum, 84
aromatherapy, 100–1
Asian women, menopause,
    111–13
atypical hyperplasia, 39

## B

balm, 80
Barlow, Prof. D H, 49
benign breast disease, 38–9
bergamot, 101
birth control pills, 12, 25, 37
bisphosphonates, 49
black cohosh, 80, 82
blood clots, 54, 58
BMA see British Medical
Association
Body Mass Index (BMI), 56
bowel cancer, 25, 42–3
BRCA2 gene, 39
breast cancer, 35–9
British Medical Association
    (BMA), 74

## C

calcitonins, 50
calcium, 46–8, 50, 112–13,
    116, 117
calorie counting, 124
cancer
    bowel, 25, 42–3
    breast, 35–9
    ovarian, 20
candle gazing, 91
carbohydrates, 107–8
cardiovascular disease (CVD), 25,
    53–9
castor oil, 78, 79
cat stretch, 135
change see menopause
chasteberry, 80
CHD see coronary heart disease
China Diet Study, 111–13
Chinese herbal medicines, 77
cholesterol, 41, 53, 54, 112

chromium, 116
clary sage, 101
climacteric, 17
    see also menopause
clinical trials
    acupuncture, 75
    breast cancer, 35
    Chinese herbal medicines, 77
    homoeopathy, 84
    massage, 96
    reflexology, 98
complementary medicines, 71–2
    acupuncture, 72–6
    combining medicines, 81, 85
    homoeopathy, 83–5
    medical herbalism, 78–82
    traditional Chinese medicine,
    77
complex carbohydrates, 107–8
continuous therapy, 30
contraceptive pills see birth
    control pills
coronary heart disease (CHD), 53,
    54
corticosteroids, 45
counselling, 88
creams see transdermal creams;
    vaginal creams
curvature of the spine, 44, 50,
    128
CVD see cardiovascular disease
cyclical therapy, 30
cypress, 101
cysts, 13, 27

## D

Dalton, Katherina, 15
dancing, 138
decoctions, 82
dehydroepiandrosterone (DHEA),
    12, 110
dementia, 41, 42
depression, 25
DHEA see
    dehydroepiandrosterone
diabetes mellitus, 53, 60–1
dietary factors
    Asian women, 111–13
    blood sugar, 109–11
    bowel cancer, 42–3
    breast cancer, 37
    carbohydrates, 107–8
    cardiovascular disease, 54,
    58–9
    diabetes mellitus, 53, 60–1
    fats, 108–9
    fatty acids, 108, 109, 117
    food chart, 118–21

menopause, 106–21
minerals, 116
osteoporosis, 45, 46–50
proteins, 108
supplements, 113, 117
vitamins, 115
*Dioscorea villosa*, 62–4
diosgenin, 62, 63
dual energy X-ray absorptiometry
    46

## E

eating disorders, 45
EFAs see essential fatty acids
endocrine system, 11–12, 98, 99
endometriosis, 13, 20–1, 24
endorphins, 125
epinephrine see adrenaline
essential fatty acids (EFAs), 109
essential oils, 100–1
estring, 34
estrogens see oestrogens
evening primrose oil, 109
exercise, 106, 124–38
    CVD, 55, 59, 124
    daily routines, 136–7
    dancing, 138
    diabetes, 60
    kneeling hand walk, 127
    leg swing, 126
    osteoporosis, 48, 125
    pilates stretches, 132–5
    posture, 128–31
    yoga, 93

## F

fall prevention, 51–2
family history, breast cancer, 38
fats, 108–9
fatty acids, 108, 109, 117
Female Hormone Kits, 27
fennel, 101
fertility, menopause, 17
fibroids, 13
Fitzgerald, Dr. William, 97
Fogelman, Prof. Ignac, 51
folklore, 79
follicle-stimulating hormone 11,
    19
food chart, 118–21
FSH see follicle-stimulating
    hormone

## G

genetic factors, breast cancer, 39
geranium, 101
gingko, 80
ginseng, 80

glucose, 60, 109–10
graphites, 84

## H

Hahnemann, Samuel, 83–4
hamstring stretch, 132
hatha yoga, 93
healing retreats, 102–3
heart disease see cardiovascular
    disease
Heart and Oestrogen/
    Progestogen Replacement
    Study (HERS), 57
herbal medicines, 77, 78–82
HERS see Heart and
    Oestrogen/Progestogen
    Replacement Study
high blood pressure, 41, 53, 54
Hippocratic School, 78
homoeopathy, 83–5
hormones, 10–16
    see also oestrogens;
        progesterone; testosterone
    endocrine system, 11–12
    function, 12
    imbalances, 12–13
    implants, 32–3
    ovarian, 14–15
    regulation, 16
hot flushes, 18–19
    acupuncture, 75
    evening primrose oil, 109
    reflexology, 98
    soy protein, 113
    traditional Chinese medicine,
    77
hysterectomy, 20–1, 30,
31, 61

## I

implants, 32–3
infusions, 82
insomnia, 65
insulin, 110
iron, 116
ischaemic heart disease, 58

## K

Kearns, Linda, 114
kneeling hand walk, 127
kyphosis see curvature of
    the spine

## L

lachesis, 84
lavender, 101
lay practitioners, 74, 84
Lee, Dr. John, 62–4, 66–7

leg swing, 126
lesbian retreats, 103
LH see luteinizing hormone
Linda Kearns Cake, 114
Ling, Prof. Per Henrik, 94
linolenic acid, 109
linseeds, 117
livial, 31
luteinizing hormone (LH), 11
lying down posture, 130–1

M
magnesium, 48, 116
manganese, 116
Marker, Dr. Russell, 62
massage, 94–6
medical herbalism, 78–82
medical tests, 27
meditation, 90–2
menopause, 17–19
    acupuncture, 76
    aromatherapy, 100–1
    Asian women, 111–13
    blood sugar, 110
    cardiovascular disease, 55
    complementary medicines,
        71–2
    dietary factors, 106–21
    exercise, 106, 124–38
    herbal remedies, 80, 82
    homoeopathy, 84, 85
    HRT, 27–8, 40
    massage, 95
    premature, 20, 45, 52
    progesterone role, 62–6
    reflexology, 99
    sexual activity, 87
    stress, 86–9
    symptoms, 6–7, 26
menstruation
    amenorrhoea, 13, 52
    hormone function, 13, 14, 15
    osteoporosis, 45
    pre-menstrual syndrome, 15,
        66, 71
    puberty, 14
mental imagery, 89
meridians, 73
Million Women Study, The, 37
minerals, 116
mood swings, 25
Mulimen, 84

N
nasal sprays, 33
National Centre for
    Complementary and
    Alternative Medicine
    (NCCAM), 72
natural oestrogen, 25
natural progesterone, 62–6

neck stretch, 134
neurotransmitters, 41

O
obesity, 54, 56, 58
oestrogens, 11
    breast cancer, 37
    endometriosis, 24
    function, 14
    HRT preparations, 25, 30–4
omega oils, 108, 109
oophorectomy, 20–1, 61
opium, 78
orthodox medicines, 85
osteoporosis, 25, 44–52, 60,
    62–3
ovarian cancer, 20
ovarian cysts, 13
ovarian hormones, 14–15
ovaries, 11, 12
    removal, 20–1
ovulation, 14, 17

P
pain relief, acupuncture, 72
pancreas, 11, 12
parathyroid glands, 11
Pasteur, Louis, 79
patches see transdermal patches
pattern of disharmony, 73, 76
Peat, Dr. Ray, 62
peri-menopause, 17, 18, 65, 80
peripheral arterial disease, 53
phosphorus, 116
phyto-oestrogens, 113–14
pilates, 128, 132–5
Pilates, Joseph, 128
pituitary gland, 11
placebo effects, 71, 77, 98
PMS see pre-menstrual syndrome
polycystic ovaries, 13
post-menopause, 17, 40
posture, 90–1, 128–31
potassium, 116
pre-menstrual syndrome (PMS),
    15, 66, 71
pregnancy
    oestrogens, 14
    progesterone, 15
premature menopause, 20, 45,
    52
preparations
    herbal medicines, 81, 82
    homoeopathy, 84
    HRT, 25, 30–4, 64–6, 67
prescription drugs, 71
private retreats, 103
progesterone, 14–15, 62–6
progestogen, 24, 25
prostaglandins, 108
proteins, 108

psychosocial factors, 86–9
puberty, 14
pulsatilla, 84

R
raw plant materials, 81
re-modelling, 44
red blood cells, 115
red clover isoflavone, 113
reflex action, 96
reflexology, 97–9
regulations, 71–2, 74, 82
relaxation methods, 88–103
    aromatherapy, 100–1
    massage, 94–6
    meditation, 90–2
    reflexology, 97–9
    retreats, 102–3
    visualization, 89
    yoga, 93
Remifemin, 82
retreats, 102–3
reverse puberty, 18

S
St John's wort, 80
saliva tests, 27
salvia, 84
saponins, 62
saturated fats, 108
selective oestrogen receptor
    modulators (SERMs), 49
selenium, 116
self-examination, 36
self-healing concept, 73
SERMs see selective oestrogen
    receptor modulators
serotonin, 41
sex hormones see androgens;
oestrogens
sexual activity
    exercise, 136
    menopause, 87
    oestrogens, 14
    progesterone, 63
    testosterone, 16, 66, 67
    vaginal creams, 33–4
shoulder stretch, 133
side-effects
    herbal medicines, 80, 82
    homoeopathy, 85
    HRT, 24, 25, 28–9, 35–9
    prescription drugs, 71
    progesterone, 66
    testosterone, 67
simple carbohydrates, 107–8
sitting posture, 130
smoking, 45, 58
sodium, 116
soy-extract tablets, 113
soya products, 113

standing posture, 129–30
stress, 86–8, 96
stretching, 93, 131–5
sulphur, 116
sunlight, 45, 48
supplements, 113, 117
surgical procedures
    endometriosis, 20–1
    hormone implants, 32–3
    hysterectomy, 20–1, 61
    oophorectomy, 20–1, 61
symptom chart, menopause, 26
synthetic oestrogen, 25

T
tension, 92
testosterone, 16, 66–7
thyroid gland, 11
thyroxine (T4), 11
tibolone, 31–2
traditional Chinese medicine, 77
transdermal creams, 14, 67
transdermal patches, 31–2
types of HRT, 30–4

U
UK Medicines Act 1968, 80
unlicensed products, 82
unsaturated fats, 109

V
vaginal creams, 33–4, 66
vaginal rings, 34
valerian, 80
varicose veins, 57, 58
venous thromboembolic disease,
    57, 58
visualization, 89
vitamins, 45, 48, 50, 58, 115

W
weight gain, 29
wild yam, 62–4
Wilson, Dr. Robert, 24

Y
yin/yang, 73–4
yoga, 93

Z
zinc, 116
zone therapy, 97

# Acknowledgements

Acestock Ltd 22 bottom left, 41, 58.

Alamy/Phoebe Dunn 8-9 bottom right, 14, /Image Source 2 centre, 7, 22 centre, 28, /Imagestate 122 top centre, 131, /Peter Mumford 68-69 bottom right, 93.

Bubbles/Jennie Woodcock 57.

Getty Images/Samuel Ashfield 37, /Ron Chapple 8 centre, /Chris Cheadle 103, /Jim Cummins 2 top left, 48, /Candice Farmer 2-3 top right, 122 centre left, 137, /Howard Grey 8 bottom centre, 13, /David Hanover 87, /Walter Hodges 122 bottom centre, 124, /Romilly Lockyer 122 top left, 125, /Stuart McClymont 2 bottom centre, 138, /Laurence Monneret 8-9 top right, 18, 22 top left, 24, /Antony Nagelmann 68 centre, 102, /Andreas Pollok 68-69, 88, /Anne Rippy 8 bottom left, 65, /Mark Scott 104-105 centre right, 106, /Steve Smith 56, /V.C.L. 27, /Terry Vine 8 centre left, 15, /Mel Yates 100.


Octopus Publishing Group Limited /Colin Bowling 2 bottom left, 62, 77, 82 centre left, 82 bottom right, /Colin Bowling /Organon Laboratories Ltd. 23 bottom right, 30, 32 centre right, 34 left, /Colin Bowling / Pharmacia Corporation 34 right, /Colin Bowling /Schering Health Care Ltd. 22 centre left,  31 centre right,
/Jean Cazals 105 top centre, 120 left, /Colin Gotts 129, /Sandra Lane 104 top right, 116, /Sean Myers 83,
/Peter Pugh-Cook 3 centre right, 9 centre right, 10, 23 top right, 59, 68 bottom left, 94, 97, 128 left, 128 right, /William Reavell 2 top centre, 2 centre left, 23 centre right, 60, 92, 101, 104 top left, 104 centre left, 104 centre, 104 bottom left, 104 bottom centre, 105 bottom right, 107, 108 right, 111, 112 top, 117, /Gareth Sambidge 66, 68 centre left, 69 centre right, 95 top left, 95 centre right, 95 bottom left, /Nikki Sianni 8 top left, 70, 90, 122 centre, 122 bottom left, 123 centre right, 126 top, 126 centre, 126 bottom, 127 centre left, 127 top right, 127 bottom right, 130, /Ian Wallace 3 bottom right, 68 top centre, 91, 99 top, 99 centre, 108 left, 112 bottom, 118 left, 118 right, 119 left, 120 right, /Philip Webb 119 right, /Mark Winwood 123 top right, 123 bottom right, 132 top right, 132 bottom left, 133 top left, 133 centre right, 133 bottom left, 134 centre left, 134 top right, 134 bottom centre, 135 top left, 135 bottom right.

Image State 136 left.

Science Photo Library/David Gifford 50, /Tim Malon & Paul Biddle 74, /Jerry Mason 32 bottom right, /Andrew McClenaghan 75, /Will & Deni McIntyre 22 top centre, 46, /Professors P.M. Motta & J. Van Blerkom 8 top right, 17, /Perlstein, Jerrican 1, 136 right, /Sinclair Stammers 22 centre bottom, 44, /Tek Image 68 top left, 72, /Sheila Terry 31 bottom right, 68 bottom centre, 78, /Th Foto-Werbung 79, /Jim Varney 55, /Hattie Young 61.

Wellfoods Limited/tel: +44 (0) 1226 381 712/ www.bake-it.com 114.

Executive Editor: **Jane McIntosh**
Managing Editor: **Clare Churly**
Design Manager: **Tokiko Morishima**
Designer: **Ruth Hope**
Senior Production Controller: **Jo Sim**
Picture Researcher: **Zoë Holtermann**
Illustrations: **Philip Wilson and Cactus Design and Illustration**